Keto Diet for Beginners Bundle

Book 1:

Ketogenic Diet for Beginners:

A Diet of Low Carb Recipes for Weight Loss

Free Gift Included

As part of our commitment to making sure you live a healthy lifestyle, we have included a free e-book in the link below. This book informs of the food groups and food items that will enable you to lose weight quickly. I hope that you enjoy this e-book and the extra gift as well. The link to the gift is below:

http://36potentfoodstoloseweightandlivehealthy.gr8.com

Disclaimer

About the author

Sam Kuma is passionate about sharing his culinary experience to the world. His work involves modernization of healthy diet plans. He has written/published books for vegan food, ketogenic food, paleo food, dash food and several foods from other ethnic cuisines. His main focus is to make healthy diets like vegan and ketogenic mainstream by producing delicious, appetizing recipes. In his first two books regarding Vegan recipes, he has produced delicious Vegan Chocolate meals, Vegan Desserts, Vegan Ice Creams, Vegan Burgers and Sandwiches.

Book description

This book is a guide for all those who want to follow the Ketogenic Diet, but have no clue where to begin. It contains detailed information as to what the Ketogenic Diet is, the do's and don'ts of the diet and a bunch of recipes that will help you kick-start your journey!

This book is full of Ketogenic Diet-friendly recipes for a variety of meals, such as soups, salads, side dishes, main courses, Ketogenic snacks and last, but not least, desserts!

All the recipes in this book are quick and easy to prepare and you will not need to spend hours in the kitchen. All the ingredients in the recipes are easily available and you do not need to go hunting for expensive specialized ingredients!

With this bunch of Ketogenic Diet-friendly recipes, you can easily and quickly pick up the diet without having to do any calorie calculations or gram-by-gram portion measurements!

This book is one-stop for all your Ketogenic Diet queries!

Table of Contents

Introduction

In a world obsessed with size zero, it seems every person with an ounce of extra weight wants to lose it. Capitalizing on this trend, a lot of "dieticians" and "nutritionists" have come up with a variety of "specialized diets" where you consume "special foods" and lose weight. All this is just a sham!

The reality is that most of the time, these "specialists" have deals with manufacturing companies, and they push the "special" products produced by companies in your face to earn a hefty commission. At the end of these diets all you will have lost is money! But, what if I tell you that there is a diet in which you do not need to purchase expensive specialized products (nor starve) and you can still lose weight without messing up your regular schedule?

Here I present to you the "**Ketogenic Diet**".

The Ketogenic Diet is quite popular, as it is a low-carb diet. The body usually converts carbohydrates to glucose and insulin. Glucose is the most basic and easiest energy source the body can break down and use to provide energy. This is why your body will ignore all sources of energy as long as there is glucose in your system. This results in deposits of fat in the body, because your body stores all the fat from your food for future use.

So, the basic idea of the Ketogenic Diet is to induce the body into a state of *ketosis* by eliminating all carbohydrate-rich foods from the diet. Ketosis is the natural state of the body where the body initiates metabolic processes to deal with the low intake of carbohydrates (and glucose). The body starts producing ketones in the liver by breaking down fat in the body.

While following the Ketogenic Diet, you stop all carbohydrate intake and up your fat intake, resulting in the production of fat-breaking ketones! This breakdown of body fat results in a leaner body!

To start following the Ketogenic Diet, you need to plan ahead and have a diet plan waiting on hand. Whatever you eat has a great impact on how fast your body attains the state of *ketosis*. The lower the carbs that you consume in a day (**preferably less than 15 grams**) the faster your body attains the state of ketosis and the quicker you will lose weight!

Your nutrient intake should be as follows:

- 70% of total nutritional content should be fat
- 25% of total nutritional content should be protein
- 5% of total nutritional content should be carbohydrates

The 5% of carbs should come mostly from dairy, nuts and vegetables, and refined carbs from cereals such as wheat, fruits or starchy vegetables such as potatoes, should be avoided.

An ideal meal should consist of the main protein meal with two sides – one full of veggies and one fat-rich. For example, a meal could consist of a grilled rib-eye steak with a knob of butter and a side of spinach stir fried in olive oil or a whole skinless and boneless chicken breast fried in very little olive oil with a side of stir-fried broccoli and cheese.

So, as you can see, this diet aids in the reduction of body fat and helps you to lose weight.

This book contains healthy Ketogenic recipes for all of your meals, from breakfast till dinner and for all courses, from soups to salads to main courses to snacks and desserts! And the best part? All of these recipes are quick and easy and use ingredients easily available in every kitchen and pantry!

I would like to thank you for purchasing this book and I hope you find the content of this book helpful!

Ketogenic Breakfast Recipes

Spicy Shrimp Omelet

Prep: 10 min	Total: 20 min	Servings: 2

Ingredients:

- 3 eggs, whisked
- 2 grape tomatoes, halved
- 1 medium onion, chopped
- 5 shrimp, peeled, deveined
- 1 tablespoon fresh parsley, chopped
- 1/4 teaspoon cayenne pepper
- 1/8 teaspoon pepper powder
- 1/4 teaspoon salt or to taste
- 1 tablespoon coconut oil
- A dash of hot sauce

Method:

1. Place a nonstick pan over medium heat. Add oil. When the oil is hot enough, add onions and sauté until onions are translucent.
2. Add salt, pepper, cayenne pepper, shrimp and tomatoes. Sauté for a couple of minutes.
3. Pour whisked eggs over it. Sprinkle parsley. Cook until the eggs are set.

4. Drizzle hot sauce over it and serve.

Raspberry Pancakes

Prep: 10 min	Total: 25 min	Servings: 2

Ingredients:

- 1 banana, mashed
- 1/2 cup egg whites, beaten
- 6 tablespoons almond milk
- 1 1/2 cup raspberries, frozen
- 1 tablespoon cinnamon
- 2 tablespoons chia seeds, ground
- 2 scoops whey powder
- Cooking spray with olive oil
- 4 tablespoons Greek yogurt to serve

Method:

1. Mix together all the ingredients, except raspberries, until well-combined.
2. Add raspberries and mix again.
3. Place a nonstick pan over medium heat. Spray with olive oil.
4. Pour about 1/4 cup mixture into the pan. Swirl the pan so that the batter spreads. Cook until the bottom side is golden brown.
5. Flip sides. Cook the other side until golden brown.
6. Repeat steps 4 and 5 with the remaining batter.
7. Serve hot with Greek yogurt.

Mock McGriddle Casserole

Prep: 10	Total: 1 hr. 10 min	Servings: 4

Ingredients:

- 5 large eggs
- 2 tablespoons butter
- 1/2-pound breakfast sausages
- 3 tablespoons maple syrup or to taste
- 1/2 teaspoon garlic powder
- 1 teaspoon onion powder
- 2 ounces' cheddar cheese
- 2 tablespoons flaxseed meal
- 1/2 cup almond flour
- Salt to taste
- Pepper powder to taste
- 1/4 teaspoon sage

Method:

1. Place a pan over medium heat. Add sausages and cook until brown and slightly crispy. Remove from heat.
2. Meanwhile, mix together in a large bowl, almond flour, flaxseed meal, salt, pepper, sage, onion and garlic powder.
3. Mix together in another bowl, 2 tablespoons maple syrup and eggs and whisk well. Pour this mixture into the almond flour mixture.
4. Add cheese and stir.

5. Pour this mixture into the pan of sausages and stir. Transfer into a lined casserole dish.
6. Drizzle the remaining tablespoon of maple syrup over it.
7. Place in a preheated oven and bake at 350°F for about 45 minutes or until cooked. A toothpick when inserted in the center should come out clean.
8. Remove from the oven and cool. Chop into wedges and serve.

Meat Bagel

Prep: 5 min	Total: 55 min	Servings: 4

Ingredients:

- 1-pound ground pork
- 1 medium onion, finely chopped
- 1 large egg
- 1/3 cup tomato sauce
- 1/2 tablespoon butter or ghee
- 1/2 teaspoon paprika
- 1/4 teaspoon pepper powder
- 1/2 teaspoon salt
- Toppings of your choice

Method:

1. Place a skillet over medium heat. Add ghee or butter. When it melts, add onions and sauté until translucent. Remove from heat and cool completely.
2. Transfer into a bowl and add rest of the ingredients and mix well.
3. Divide into 3 or 4 equal portions and shape into a bagel.
4. Place in a baking dish that is lined with parchment paper.
5. Bake in a preheated oven at 400°F for about 40 minutes or until done.
6. Slice the bagels. Fill with toppings of your choice and serve.

Breakfast Cereal Mix

Prep: 5 min	Total: 10 min	Servings: 4

Ingredients:

- 10 tablespoons coconut flakes, unsweetened
- 14 tablespoons hemp seeds
- 10 tablespoons flaxseed, ground
- 4 tablespoons sesame, ground (grind for just a few seconds)
- 4 tablespoons dark cocoa, unsweetened
- 4 tablespoons psyllium husk
- 1 cup almonds, chopped

Method:

1. Mix together all the ingredients and place in an airtight container. Refrigerate until use.
2. To serve, add water or coffee or any non-dairy milk, soak for a while and serve.

Avocado Breakfast Bowl

Prep: 5 min	Total: 5 min	Servings: 4

Ingredients:

- 2 large avocados, peeled, pitted, halved
- 4 tablespoons tahini
- 1 large carrot, shredded

For dressing:
- 2 tablespoons lemon juice
- 2 tablespoons extra virgin olive oil
- 1/2 teaspoons ginger, grated
- 1/2 tablespoons poppy seeds
- 1/8 teaspoon salt

Method:

1. Whisk together all the ingredients of the dressing and carrots.
2. Fill the avocado halves with mixture.
3. Top with tahini and serve.
4. Scoop along with the avocado and eat.

Skillet-Baked Eggs

Prep: 10 min	Total: 40 min	Servings: 6

Ingredients:

- 1 cup plain Greek yogurt
- 2 cloves garlic, halved
- Kosher salt to taste
- 3 tablespoons unsalted butter, divided
- 3 tablespoons olive oil
- 5 tablespoons leek, chopped, white and pale green part only
- 3 tablespoons scallions, chopped, white and pale green parts only
- 15 ounces' fresh spinach, rinsed
- 2 teaspoons fresh lemon juice
- 6 large eggs
- 1/2 teaspoon crushed red pepper flakes
- 1/4 teaspoon paprika
- 2 teaspoons fresh oregano, chopped

Method:

1. To a small bowl, add yogurt, garlic and a pinch of salt. Mix well and keep aside.
2. Place a skillet over medium heat. Add half the butter. When butter melts, add leeks and scallions.
3. Lower the heat. Cook until softened.
4. Add spinach, salt and lemon juice.

5. Increase the heat to medium/high. Sauté for a few minutes until the spinach is wilted.
6. Transfer the contents to a large ovenproof dish. Do not add the excess liquid that is present in the spinach mixture.
7. Make 6 wells or cavities in the mixture.
8. Gently break an egg into each of the wells.
9. Place the dish in a preheated oven. Bake at 300°F until the eggs are set.
10. Place a small saucepan over medium-low heat. Add the remaining butter. When the butter melts, add the yogurt mixture and a pinch of salt. Cook for a few seconds and add oregano. Cook for 20-30 seconds and remove from heat. Discard the garlic halves.
11. Pour the yogurt mixture over the eggs and serve.

Cheese Muffins

Prep: 10 min	Total: 40min	Servings: 8

Ingredients:

- 1 cup almond flour
- 1/4 teaspoon baking soda
- A pinch salt
- 1/4 teaspoon dried thyme
- 1 egg, beaten
- 1/2 cup sour cream
- 1 tablespoon butter, melted
- 1/2 cup cheddar cheese, shredded
- 1/4 cup muenster cheese, shredded

Method:

1. Place cupcake papers in the muffin molds.
2. Mix together almond flour, salt, and baking soda in a bowl.
3. In a large bowl add butter, egg, and sour cream. Mix well. Add the almond flour mixture and mix well. If the batter is too thick add a little water or some more sour cream. Add cheese and mix well.
4. Pour into the muffin molds (fill up to 2/3).
5. Bake in a preheated oven at 350°F for about 20 minutes or until golden. A toothpick when inserted in the center should come out clean.
6. Remove from the oven and cool. Serve topped with butter.

Chocolate Smoothie

Prep: 5 min	Total: 7min	Servings: 2

Ingredients:

- 2 cups, almond milk, unsweetened
- Few drops stevia of honey or agave nectar any other artificial sweetener to taste
- 1/2 cup heavy cream
- 3 scoops chocolate flavored whey powder

Method:

1. Place all the ingredients into a blender and blend until smooth and creamy.
2. Pour into tall glasses.
3. Serve immediately with crushed ice.

Green Smoothie

Prep: 5 min	Total: 7 min	Servings: 2

Ingredients:

- 4 cups spinach
- 2 cups coconut milk, chilled, unsweetened
- 4 Brazil nuts
- 2/3 cup almonds
- 2 tablespoons psyllium husk
- 2 scoops whey protein powder
- 2 scoops greens powder
- 4 drops stevia or to taste (optional)

Method:

1. Place spinach, almonds, Brazil nuts and coconut milk into a blender and blend until smooth.
2. Add rest of the ingredients and blend until smooth and creamy.
3. Pour into tall glasses.
4. Serve immediately with crushed ice.

Berry Chocolate Shake

Prep: 5 min	Total: 7 min	Servings: 2

Ingredients:

- 2 cups almond milk
- 1/2 cup blueberries / blackberries / strawberries / raspberries
- 1/4 cup cocoa powder
- Stevia drops to taste
- 1/2 teaspoon xanthan gum
- 2 tablespoons MCT oil
- Few ice cubes

Method:

1. Blend together all the ingredients until smooth.
2. Pour into tall glasses and serve.

Matcha Smoothie Bowl

Prep: 5 min	Total: 7 min	Servings: 2

Ingredients:

- 2 tablespoons goji berries
- 2 teaspoons matcha powder
- 2 tablespoons cacao nibs
- 2 tablespoons chia seeds
- 2 tablespoons coconut flakes
- 2 tablespoons chia seeds
- 2 cups coconut yogurt or full-fat Greek yogurt
- 2 scoops greens powder (optional)

Method:

1. Add matcha powder, greens powder if using and yogurt to a blender and blend until smooth.
2. Pour into 2 individual bowls. Add the rest of the ingredients to the mixture.
3. Stir, chill for a while and serve.

Healthy Smoothie

Prep: 10 min	Total: 12 min	Servings: 4

Ingredients:

- 1 cup frozen strawberries
- 1 cup frozen raspberries
- 1 cup frozen blueberries
- 1 cup frozen blackberries
- 2 cups kale, stems and tough ribs removed, roughly chopped
- 2 cups spinach
- 1 cup orange segments
- 1 cup water
- 1/2 cup soft tofu

Method:

1. Place all the ingredients into a blender and blend until smooth and creamy.
2. Pour into tall glasses.
3. Serve

Ketogenic Soup Recipes

Chicken Enchilada Soup

Prep: 15 min	Total: 45 min	Servings: 8

Ingredients:

- 2 tablespoons olive oil
- 6 stalks celery, chopped
- 2 medium red bell pepper, chopped
- 4 teaspoons garlic, minced
- 8 cups chicken broth
- 2 cups tomatoes, chopped
- 2 cups cream cheese
- 12 ounces' chicken, cooked, shredded
- 1 1/2 tablespoons ground cumin
- 2 teaspoons oregano
- 2 teaspoons chili powder
- 1 teaspoon cayenne pepper
- 1 cup cilantro, chopped
- Juice of a lime

Method:

1. Place a large pot over medium heat. Add oil. When the oil is heated, add celery and bell pepper. Sauté until the celery is softened.
2. Add tomatoes and sauté for a couple of minutes.

3. Add cumin, oregano, chili powder and cayenne pepper. Mix well.
4. Add chicken broth and cilantro. Bring to the boil.
5. Lower heat and simmer for about 20 minutes.
6. Add cream cheese. Mix well and bring to the boil. Simmer again for about 30 minutes.
7. Add lime juice, mix well and garnish with cilantro.
8. Ladle soup into individual soup bowls and serve hot.

Spanish Sardine and Tomato Soup

Prep: 10 min	Total: 30 min	Servings: 8

Ingredients:

- 9 ounces canned Spanish sardines in tomato sauce and olive oil
- 2 tablespoons olive oil
- 2 large tomatoes, sliced
- 4 cups fresh spinach
- 2 onions, sliced
- 2 cloves garlic, sliced
- 1 teaspoon black pepper powder
- 1 1/2 teaspoons salt or to taste
- 6 cups water

Method:

1. Place a large pot over medium heat. Add oil. When the oil is heated, add onions and garlic. Sauté until onions are softened.
2. Add tomatoes and sauté for a few minutes until tomatoes are soft.
3. Add sardines and sauté for a few minutes crushing the sardines simultaneously.
4. Add water and bring to the boil.
5. Lower heat and add spinach, salt and pepper. Let it simmer until spinach wilts.
6. Ladle soup into individual soup bowls and serve hot.

Hot Chili Soup

Prep: 10 min	Total: 45 min	Servings: 4

Ingredients:

- 12 ounces' chicken thighs
- 3 cups chicken broth
- 3 tablespoons olive oil
- 3 tablespoons butter
- 6 tablespoons tomato paste
- 3 cups water
- 2 teaspoons coriander seeds
- 3 chili peppers, sliced
- 1 teaspoon ground turmeric
- 1 large avocado, peeled, pitted, sliced
- 3 chili pepper sliced or to taste
- 1 teaspoon ground cumin
- 3 ounces Queso fresco cheese
- 3 tablespoons lime juice
- Salt to taste
- Pepper powder to taste

Method:

1. Place chicken in a skillet. Sprinkle salt and pepper over it. Pour about one tablespoon oil over it and coat well.
2. Place the skillet over medium heat. Cook until chicken is tender. Place chicken thighs into individual soup bowls.

3. Place skillet back on heat. Add remaining oil. When oil is heated, add coriander seeds and sauté for a few seconds until fragrant.
4. Add chili pepper and sauté for a few seconds. Add water and bring to the boil. Add salt, pepper, turmeric, and ground cumin.
5. Reduce heat and let it simmer. Add tomato paste and butter and continue simmering for another 10 minutes.
6. Pour soup over chicken.
7. Place a few slices of avocado in each bowl, a little Queso fresco cheese and cilantro and serve.

Chilled Avocado Soup

Prep: 5 min	Total: 7 min	Servings: 6

Ingredients:

- 3 cups Hass avocado puree
- 3 cups vegetable broth
- 3 cups heavy cream
- 1/2 cup cilantro, chopped
- 2 jalapeno peppers, deseeded, chopped
- 2 teaspoons ground cumin
- 1 teaspoon salt or to taste

Method:

1. Add all the ingredients to a food processor and blend until smooth.
2. Chill until use.
3. Serve in individual bowls.

Light Zucchini Soup

Prep: 5 min	Total: 25 min	Servings: 3

Ingredients:

- 1 medium zucchini, chopped into cubes
- 2 cups vegetable stock
- 1 small onion, chopped
- 1 small chili pepper, chopped
- Salt to taste
- Pepper
- 1/4 cup fresh dill, chopped
- 1 tablespoon olive oil

Method:

1. Place a pot over medium heat. Add oil. When the oil is heated, add onions and pepper. Sauté until onions are translucent.
2. Add stock, salt, and pepper. Simmer for 8-10 minutes. Add zucchini and simmer further until tender. Remove from heat.
3. Add dill and serve either hot or cold. For cold, chill in the refrigerator.

Cream of Broccoli Soup

Prep: 15 min	Total: 30 min	Servings: 6

Ingredients:

- 1 large cauliflower, broken into florets
- 6 cups broccoli, finely chopped
- 2 yellow onions, sliced
- 2 teaspoons extra virgin olive oil
- 5 cups almond milk, unsweetened
- 1 1/2 teaspoons sea salt
- Freshly ground black pepper
- 2 tablespoons onion powder

Method:

1. Place a large saucepan over medium heat. Add oil. When oil is heated, add onions and sauté until translucent. Season with salt, pepper, cauliflower and milk. Stir and bring to the boil.
2. Lower heat and cover, and simmer until soft. Add half the broccoli and remove from heat. Cool for a while.
3. Add to a blender and blend until smooth. Transfer it back to the saucepan.
4. Add remaining half broccoli and onion powder and stir. Place the saucepan back on heat and simmer until broccoli is tender.

Cream of Mushroom Soup

Prep: 15 min	Total: 30 min	Servings: 6

Ingredients:

- 1 tablespoon butter
- 1/2 cup carrots, diced
- 1 onions thinly sliced
- 2 teaspoons garlic, minced
- 1/4 teaspoons dried thyme or oregano
- 1/4 teaspoon black pepper powder
- 3/4 pound white mushrooms, sliced
- 4 cups vegetable broth
- 1/2 cup water
- 1 cup almond milk
- 1 green onion, thinly sliced

Method:

1. Place a heavy saucepan over medium heat. Add butter. When butter melts, add onion and garlic and sauté for a couple of minutes. Add thyme and pepper, sauté until the onions are light brown.
2. Add mushrooms, sauté for a minute. Add broth, and water and boil.
3. Remove about 1/2 a cup of vegetables from the soup and keep aside.
4. Blend the remaining soup with a stick blender.

5. Pour the blended soup back to the saucepan. Return to heat. Add milk and the retained vegetables. Simmer for about 5 minutes or until thoroughly heated.
6. Garnish with sliced green onion and serve hot.

Ketogenic Salad Recipes

Tuna Salad

Prep: 15 min	Total: 16 min	Servings: 2

Ingredients:

- 1 cup canned tuna
- 2 cups crunchy lettuce
- 1 hardboiled egg, chopped
- 1 spring onion, chopped
- 1 tablespoon lemon juice
- Pink Himalayan salt
- 1 tablespoon low-carb mayonnaise

Method:

1. Mix together all the ingredients in a bowl and toss well.
2. Serve.

Cold Chicken Salad

Prep: 10 min	Total: 40	Servings: 3-4

Ingredients:

- 6 chicken tenders
- 1 onion, chopped
- 4 radishes, halved
- 1 tablespoon fresh dill, chopped
- 1 stalk celery, chopped
- 1/2 cup mayonnaise
- 1 teaspoon salt
- 1 teaspoon pepper powder
- 1/4 cup minced dill pickle
- Cooking spray

Method:

1. Place the chicken in a greased baking dish and bake at 350°F until done.
2. Place radish in another baking dish and spray with cooking spray. Place in the oven and bake until done.
3. Remove from oven and cool. Chop radish into smaller pieces and place in a serving dish.
4. Add chicken and rest of the ingredients to it and toss well.
5. Chill for a while and serve.

Egg and Avocado Salad

Prep: 15 min	Total: 16 min	Servings: 6-8

Ingredients:

- 8 large eggs, hard-boiled, quartered
- 2 large avocados, peeled, pitted, sliced
- 2 tablespoons extra virgin olive oil
- 8 cups mixed lettuce, rinsed
- 4 cloves garlic, crushed
- 1 cup full fat yogurt or 1/2 cup low-carb mayonnaise
- 2 teaspoons Dijon mustard
- 2 tablespoons fresh chives
- 2 tablespoons basil, chopped
- 2 tablespoons thyme, chopped
- Salt to taste
- Pepper powder to taste

Method:

1. To make dressing: Mix together yogurt, garlic, Dijon mustard and salt and pepper in a bowl.
2. Place salad greens and dressing in a serving bowl and mix well. Layer with avocados followed by eggs. Sprinkle salt and pepper and serve.

Tri Color Salad

Prep: 7 min	Total: 8 min	Servings: 6

Ingredients:

- 7-8 medium tomatoes, sliced
- 2 large avocados, seeded, peeled, sliced
- 10 olives, sliced
- 1 cup mozzarella, cubed
- 1/4 cup pesto
- 1/4 cup extra virgin olive oil
- Salt to taste
- Pepper powder to taste
- 2 tablespoons fresh basil, chopped

Method:

1. Add all the ingredients to a large bowl. Toss well and serve.

Caper and Lemon Salad

Prep: 5 min	Total: 15 min	Servings: 8-10

Ingredients:

- 3 pounds' salmon fillet
- Salt to taste
- Pepper to taste
- Juice of a lemon or to taste
- 1 teaspoon lemon zest, grated
- 1/3 cup canned capers, drained, rinsed
- 3 stalks celery, chopped
- 3 teaspoons fresh dill, chopped
- 3 tablespoons extra virgin olive oil

Method:

1. Season the salmon with salt and pepper and bake in a preheated oven at 350 °F for 10 minutes or until the salmon is flaky. Let it cool for a while.
2. Transfer the salmon to a serving bowl. Add lemon juice and zest, capers, celery, dill and olive oil and toss well
3. Place in the refrigerator until use.

Salmon, Bacon and Kale Salad

Prep: 15 min	Total: 25 min	Servings: 6

Ingredients:

- 1 1/2 pounds' salmon fillets, skinless
- 2 bunches kale, discard hard ribs and stems, torn
- 8 slices bacon
- 1 cup almonds, sliced
- 1 medium red onion, thinly sliced
- 4 tablespoons lemon juice
- 1/2 cup olive oil
- Salt to taste
- Pepper powder to taste

Method:

1. Sprinkle salt and pepper over the salmon. Place the fillets on a broiler pan and place the pan in a preheated oven.
2. Bake at 425°F for 15 -18 minutes or until salmon flakes easily when pricked with a fork. Remove from oven and set aside for a while.
3. Meanwhile, place a skillet over medium heat. Add bacon and cook until crisp. Remove from pan. When cool enough to handle, crumble the bacon.
4. When salmon cools, break into flakes and add to a large serving dish. Add kale, bacon, onions and almonds. Toss well.

5. In a small bowl, whisk together oil and lemon juice. Pour over the salad, toss well and serve.

Thai Salad

Prep: 15 min	Total: 16 min	Servings: 3-4

Ingredients:

- 1/2 cup carrots, peeled, chopped
- 1/4 cup cilantro, chopped
- 1 clove garlic, minced
- Juice of 1/2 a lemon
- 1 1/2 cups kale, chopped
- 1 cup Napa cabbage, chopped
- 1/4 cup peanuts, roasted, unsalted
- 1 red bell pepper, chopped
- 1 cup thin coconut milk
- 2 tablespoons creamy peanut butter
- 1/2 teaspoon Sriracha sauce
- 1/2 teaspoon yellow curry powder
- Kosher salt to taste

Method:

1. Mix together all the ingredients in a large bowl and toss well.
2. Serve.

Ketogenic Main Course Recipes

Spicy Chicken Nuggets

Prep: 10 min	Total: 40 min	Servings: 4

Ingredients:

- 1-ounce pork rinds
- 16 ounces' chicken tenders, chopped into bite-sized pieces
- 2 tablespoons almond flour
- 1 egg, beaten
- 1/4 teaspoon chili powder
- Cayenne pepper to taste
- 1/4 teaspoon garlic powder
- 1/2 teaspoon onion powder
- 1/4 teaspoon Creole seasoning
- Salt to taste
- Pepper powder to taste

Method:

1. Blend together pork rind, onion and garlic powder, Creole seasoning, almond flour, salt, pepper, chili powder and cayenne pepper in a blender. Transfer into a bowl.
2. First, dip a chicken nugget in egg and then in the almond flour mixture. Place onto a greased baking sheet. Repeat with the remaining nuggets.
3. Bake in a preheated oven at 400°F for 20 minutes or until brown and crisp.

Chicken in Butter Gravy

Prep: 10 min	Total: 45 min	Servings: 4

Ingredients:

- 1 1/2 pounds' chicken thighs with bones
- 1/2 cup water
- 1/2 cup pureed tomatoes
- 1/4 cup heavy cream
- 3 tablespoons butter
- 1/2 tablespoon olive oil
- 1 teaspoon coconut oil
- 3/4 teaspoon ginger paste
- 3/4 teaspoon garlic paste
- 1/2 teaspoon coriander, ground
- Salt to taste
- 1/2 teaspoon garam masala powder (Indian spice blend)
- 1/4 teaspoon Kashmiri chili powder
- 1/2 teaspoon paprika
- 1/2 teaspoon red chili powder
- Cilantro for garnishing, chopped
- Cauliflower rice to serve - refer to chapter 5

Method:

1. Rub the chicken thighs with olive oil, salt, and pepper. Keep aside for 15-20 minutes.

2. Roast in a preheated oven at 375°F for about 25 minutes or until almost cooked (it should not be fully cooked). When almost cooked, remove from the oven, cool. Remove the bones from the pieces and keep aside.
3. Place butter and coconut oil in a medium-sized pan over medium heat.
4. When butter melts, add ginger and garlic paste. Sauté for a couple of minutes. Add tomatoes, coriander powder, chili powder, garam masala, paprika, and Kashmir chili powder. Simmer for a while until the butter is visible on top.
5. Add the chicken pieces, cream and water and simmer for another 5 minutes.
6. Serve hot garnished with cilantro leaves and cauliflower rice.

Ground Pork Tacos

Prep: 10 min	Total: 40 min	Servings: 8

Ingredients:

- 2 pounds' ground pork
- 1 1/2 teaspoons garlic powder
- 1 1/2 teaspoons onion powder
- 1 teaspoon sea salt
- 1 teaspoon ground cumin
- 1/2 teaspoon ground pepper or to taste
- 1/4 cup salsa
- 15 large lettuce leaves or more if required
- 3/4 cup green bell pepper, chopped
- 3/4 cup red bell pepper, chopped
- 2 medium onions, chopped

Method:

1. Add pork, garlic powder, onion powder, salt, cumin, and pepper to a skillet. Mix well using your hands.
2. Place the skillet over medium heat. Stir constantly and cook until the pork is browned well.
3. Remove the pork with a slotted spoon and place in a bowl. Discard the remaining fat.
4. Add salsa and mix well. Taste and adjust the seasonings if necessary.

5. Lay the lettuce leaves on your working area. Place some pork filling in the center.
6. Sprinkle peppers, and onions. Wrap it up and serve.

Italian Pork Cutlets

Prep: 10 min	Total: 45 min	Servings: 10

Ingredients:

- 10 pork cutlets
- 3/4 cup Italian dressing
- 1/4 cup parmesan cheese, grated
- Seasoning of your choice

Method:

1. Place the Italian dressing in a bowl. Add seasoning.
2. Place the cheese in another bowl.
3. Place a skillet over medium heat. Dip the cutlets in the Italian dressing.
4. Next roll it in the cheese and place in it the pan. Cook on both the sides until brown and cooked through.
5. Serve hot with Italian low-carb salsa.

Sri Lankan Fish Curry

Prep: 10 min	Total: 40 min	Servings: 6

Ingredients:

- 6 pieces (about 2 pounds) Silver Hake or any other white fish
- 6 tablespoons coconut oil
- 1/2 teaspoon whole mustard seeds
- 3 long green chilies, deseeded, cut into small pieces
- 1/2 tablespoon fresh ginger, grated
- 1/2 teaspoon ground cumin
- 1/2 tablespoon curry powder
- 2-inch fresh turmeric root, grated or 3/4 teaspoon ground turmeric powder
- 1 red onion, finely chopped
- 5 cloves of garlic, chopped
- 2 1/2 cups full-fat coconut cream
- 1 teaspoon sea salt
- Chopped cilantro to garnish
- 3/4 cup water

Method:

1. Place a large saucepan over medium heat. Add half the coconut oil. When the oil is melted, add mustard seeds. In a while it will start sputtering. When the sound of spluttering reduces, add onions and sauté for a few minutes.
2. Add ginger and garlic. Sauté for 4-5 minutes.

3. Add green chilies, curry powder, cumin powder and turmeric. Sauté for a couple of minutes more.
4. Add coconut milk and salt. Mix well and bring to the boil.
5. Reduce heat and simmer for about 15 minutes.
6. Meanwhile, add rest of the oil to a nonstick pan. Place the pan over medium heat.
7. Add fish to it and fry for 2 -3 minutes. When the underside is cooked, flip sides and cook the other side too.
8. Add fish to the simmering curry. Simmer for 5-7 minutes.
9. Garnish with cilantro and serve.

Coconut and Shrimp Avocadoes

Prep: 10 min	Total: 20 min	Servings: 2

Ingredients:

- 1 avocado, peeled, pitted, chop into bite-sized cubes
- 2 cups shrimp
- 2 teaspoons Sriracha sauce or any other hot sauce
- 1 tablespoon natural peanut butter
- 2 teaspoons shredded coconut
- 2 tablespoons light coconut milk
- Cooking spray

Method:

1. Place a nonstick pan over medium heat. Spray with cooking spray.
2. Add coconut milk, peanut butter and hot sauce. Stir until well combined.
3. Add shrimp and cook until shrimp are tender.
4. Remove from heat and sprinkle coconut over it.
5. Place avocados on a serving plate. Place the shrimp over it and serve.

Baked Salmon

Prep: 5 min	Total: 1 hr. 50 min	Servings: 4

Ingredients:

- 4 salmon fillets (around 6 ounces each)
- 4 cloves garlic, minced
- 12 tablespoons light olive oil
- 2 teaspoons dried basil
- 1 teaspoon salt or to taste
- 1 teaspoon ground black pepper
- 2 tablespoons lemon juice
- 2 tablespoons fresh parsley, chopped

Method:

1. Mix together in a glass dish, garlic, oil, basil, salt, pepper, lemon juice, and parsley.
2. Add salmon and mix well. Place in the refrigerator to marinate for at least an hour. Turn around the salmon a couple of times in-between.
3. Transfer the salmon, along with the marinade, to aluminum foil. Seal well. Place it in an ovenproof dish and bake for about 45 minutes in a preheated oven at 375°F.
4. Remove from the oven. When cool enough to handle, unwrap and serve with a low-carb salad of your choice.

Lamb Souvlaki (Greek Lamb Skewers)

Prep: 20 min	Total: 8 hrs. 45 min	Servings: 6-8

Ingredients:

- 2 1/2 pounds' lamb, chopped into medium size pieces
- 1/2 cup fresh mint, chopped or 2 teaspoons dried mint
- 3 tablespoons fresh rosemary, chopped or 2 teaspoons dried rosemary
- Juice of 2 lemons
- 3/4 cup extra virgin olive oil
- 1 teaspoon salt or to taste
- Melitzanosalata (eggplant dip) to serve

Method:

1. Add olive oil and lemon juice to a large bowl. Add salt, mint, and rosemary and mix well.
2. Add the lamb pieces and mix well. Marinate in the refrigerator overnight. Toss it a couple of times in between or more often.
3. Thread the meat pieces onto skewers. Place the skewers on the rack in a preheated oven.
4. Roast at 450°F until done. Turn the skewers around a couple of times in-between.
5. Remove from the oven. Let it cool for a couple of minutes. Remove from the skewers.
6. Serve with Melitzanosalata.

Ground Beef and Spinach Skillet

Prep: 15 min	Total: 45 min	Servings: 3-4

Ingredients:

- 4 tablespoons coconut oil or ghee
- 2 king oyster mushrooms, chopped
- 4 tablespoons raw almonds, chopped
- 3/4-pound lean ground beef
- 1/2 teaspoon chili pepper flakes
- A large pinch of Himalayan salt
- A large pinch of ground white pepper
- 1/2 cups pitted Kalamata olives
- 2 tablespoons capers
- 2 tablespoons natural roasted almond butter
- 3/4-pound baby spinach leaves, roughly chopped

Method:

1. Place a heavy-bottomed skillet over medium high heat. Add coconut oil. When oil melts, add mushrooms and sauté until brown.
2. Add almonds and sauté for a minute. Add beef, salt, white pepper powder, chili pepper flakes and cook until the meat is brown and cooked well.
3. Add olives, capers and almond butter. Mix well. Add spinach and sauté for a couple of minutes until the spinach wilts well.
4. Serve immediately.

Low-Carb Shepherd's Pie

Prep: 10 min	Total: 1 hr. 30 min	Servings: 6-8

Ingredients:

- 2 pounds extra lean ground beef
- 2 cloves garlic, minced
- 1 large yellow onion, chopped
- 1 packet frozen vegetables
- 4 cups cauliflower florets
- 2 teaspoons steak seasoning
- 2 teaspoons black pepper powder
- Sea salt to taste
- 1 cup beef broth
- 1 cup chicken broth
- 2 teaspoons dried rosemary

Method:

1. Place a large pot of water over medium heat and add about a teaspoon of salt and cauliflower florets to it. Cook until tender. Drain and set aside to allow it to cool.
2. Mash well and set aside.
3. Place a large skillet over medium heat. Add onion, garlic, and meat. Sauté.
4. Cook until the meat is browned and keep aside.
5. Remove the meat mixture with a slotted spoon. Drain off the excess fat and add the meat mixture back to the skillet.

6. Add steak seasoning, salt, pepper, beef broth, chicken broth and frozen vegetables.
7. Cook until the excess liquid dries up.
8. Transfer this mixture into a large baking dish.
9. Spread mashed cauliflower mixture over the meat mixture.
10. Place the baking dish into a preheated oven at 350°F and bake for 20 -30 minutes or longer if you want it browner.

Spinach Pie

Prep: 10 min	Total: 1 hr.	Servings: 4

Ingredients:

- 1/4 cup butter
- 1/4 cup chopped onions
- 2 packages (16 ounces each) frozen chopped spinach, thawed, drained, squeezed of extra moisture
- 6 eggs
- 3 cups heavy cream
- 1 teaspoon salt
- 1 teaspoon black pepper powder
- 1 teaspoon ground nutmeg
- 1 cup Swiss cheese, shredded

Method:

1. Place a large saucepan over medium heat. Add most of the butter. When butter melts, add onions and sauté until the onions are translucent.
2. Add spinach. Cook until the mixture is almost dry. Transfer into a greased pie pan. Sprinkle cheese. Place blobs of remaining butter in 4-5 places.
3. Bake in a preheated oven for about 30 minutes.

Low-Carb Pad Thai

Prep: 15 min	Total: 16	Servings: 3-4

Ingredients:

- 2 packets kelp noodles
- 1 large onion, chopped
- 6 cloves garlic, minced
- 1 cup peanut butter
- 1/2 cup soy sauce or tamari
- 3 teaspoons red pepper flakes or to taste
- 1/4 cup lime juice
- 1 large carrot, peeled, shredded
- 2 scallions, chopped
- 2 tablespoons fresh cilantro, chopped
- 2 tablespoons sesame seeds, toasted

Method:

1. Place kelp noodles in a bowl and pour water over it. Set aside for it to soak.
2. Meanwhile, blend together onion, garlic, peanut butter, soy sauce, pepper flakes and lime juice until smooth.
3. When the noodles have soaked, drain the excess water.
4. Pour sauce over it. Sprinkle carrots, scallions, and cilantro and sesame seeds over it and serve.

Stir Fried Bacon & Vegetables

Prep: 20 min	Total: 30 min	Servings: 3-4

Ingredients:

- 10 strips smoked bacon, chopped into fine pieces
- 2 cups kale, discard hard stems and ribs
- 1 medium head broccoli, chopped into florets
- 1 red bell pepper, sliced
- 1 cup green beans, chopped into 1-inch pieces
- 2 small courgettes, chopped
- 2 cloves garlic, chopped
- 2 teaspoons butter
- 2 teaspoons coconut oil
- Salt to taste
- Pepper powder to taste
- 1 cup thick single cream
- Cauliflower rice to serve – refer to chapter 5

Method:

1. Place a skillet over medium heat. Add coconut oil and butter. When it melts, add garlic and sauté until fragrant.
2. Add all the vegetables, salt and pepper and sauté until the vegetables are crisp and tender as well.
3. Add bacon and stir for a couple of minutes. Remove from heat. Add cream and mix.
4. Serve over cauliflower rice.

Zucchini Casserole

Prep: 15 min	Total: 45 min	Servings: 6-8

Ingredients:

- 12 cups zucchini, diced
- 1 red bell pepper chopped
- 1 yellow bell pepper, chopped
- 1 cup quinoa, cook according to the package instructions
- 1 1/2 cups cheddar cheese, shredded
- 3/4 cup olive oil
- 1 1/2 teaspoons dried basil
- 3 eggs, beaten
- Salt to taste
- Pepper powder to taste

Method:

1. Mix together all the ingredients in a bowl. Transfer to a greased baking dish.
2. Spread the mixture all over.
3. Bake in a preheated oven at 350°F until top is golden brown.

Low-Carb Pizza

Prep: 5 min	Total: 45 min	Servings: 6-8

Ingredients:

For pizza crust:
- 6 eggs
- 26 ounces' cream cheese, softened
- 1/3 cup parmesan cheese, grated
- 3 cups mozzarella cheese, shredded
- 1/2 cup heavy cream
- 1/2 teaspoon garlic powder
- 1 teaspoon pizza seasoning
- 2 teaspoons chives

For topping:
- 3/4 cup low-carb pizza sauce or as required
- Toppings of your choice (low-carb)
- 1 1/2 cups mozzarella cheese, shredded

Method:

1. To make crust: Add cream cheese and egg to a bowl and beat well. Add heavy cream, parmesan, chives, pizza seasoning and garlic.
2. Grease a baking dish and place mozzarella cheese into it. Pour cream cheese mixture over it.
3. Bake in a preheated oven at 375°F for about 30 minutes.

4. Remove from the oven. Spread pizza sauce over it and add toppings of your choice.

Ketogenic Side Dishes

Cauliflower Garlic Breadsticks

Prep: 15 min	Total: 50 min	Servings: 4-6

Ingredients:

- 4 cups cauliflower, grated, microwaved for 3 minutes
- 2 tablespoons butter
- 6 teaspoons minced garlic
- 1/2 teaspoon red pepper flakes
- 1 teaspoon Italian seasoning
- Kosher salt to taste
- 2 cups mozzarella cheese, shredded
- 2 eggs, beaten
- 2 tablespoons parmesan cheese powder

Method:

1. Place a pan over low heat. Add butter. When butter melts, add garlic flakes and red pepper flakes and cook for 2-3 minutes.
2. Add this to cooked cauliflower. Add salt and Italian seasoning. Mix well.
3. Add beaten eggs and mozzarella cheese. Mix well.
4. Transfer the mixture to a greased baking dish. Press well. Bake in a preheated oven at 350°F for 30 minutes.
5. Remove from oven. Sprinkle some more mozzarella and Parmesan cheese.
6. Bake for another 8-10 minutes.

7. Remove from oven. Cut into sticks.
8. Serve hot with low-sugar tomato sauce.

Keto Bread / Muffins

Prep: 5 min	Total: 35 min	Servings: 8-10

Ingredients:

- 6 large eggs
- 1 cup almond flour
- 3 teaspoons baking powder
- 4 tablespoons butter

Method:

1. Add all the ingredients into a bowl. Whisk well until the batter is smooth and well aerated.
2. Transfer to a greased baking loaf pan.
3. Bake in a preheated oven at 390°F for about 20 minutes or until done.
4. If you want to make muffins, then pour the batter into greased muffin tins (fill up to 2/3).
5. Slice and serve.

Mashed Cauliflower (Mock Mashed Potatoes)

Prep: 15 min	Total: 30 min	Servings: 6-8

Ingredients:

- 3 heads cauliflower, chopped into small florets
- 6 tablespoons heavy cream
- 3 tablespoons butter
- 3/4 cup cheddar cheese, shredded
- Salt to taste
- Pepper to taste

Method:

1. Place the cauliflower florets in a microwaveable bowl along with 1 tablespoon of cream and 1 tablespoon of butter.
2. Microwave on high for 6 minutes, uncovered. Add the remaining butter and cream.
3. Mix well and microwave on high for 6-7 minutes more.
4. Remove from microwave. Add cheese and blend with an immersion blender until smooth or blend in a food processor.
5. Add salt and pepper to taste.

Mushroom and Hemp Seeds Pilaf

Prep: 10 min	Total: 25 min	Servings: 6

Ingredients:

- 2 cups hemp seeds
- 1/4 cup butter
- 6-8 mushrooms, chopped into pieces
- 1/2 cup almonds, sliced
- 1 cup broth (vegetable or chicken)
- 1 teaspoon garlic powder
- 1/2 teaspoon dried parsley
- Salt to taste
- Pepper powder to taste

Method:

1. Place a pan over medium heat. Add butter. When the butter melts, add mushrooms and almonds. Sauté for a few minutes until the mushrooms are tender.
2. Add hemp seeds and mix well. Add broth, garlic powder, parsley, salt, and pepper. Mix well.
3. Lower the heat and simmer until the broth is absorbed
4. Serve with any curry or as it is.

Cauliflower Rice

Prep: 10 min	Total: 25 min	Servings: 4-6

Ingredients:

- 2 heads cauliflower, chopped into florets
- 1 onion, finely diced
- 4 tablespoons olive oil
- 4 cloves garlic, minced
- Salt to taste
- Pepper powder to taste

Method:

1. Add the cauliflower florets to the food processor and pulse until you get a rice-like texture. You can also grate the cauliflower.
2. Place a large nonstick skillet over medium-high heat. Add oil. When oil is heated, add onions and sauté until translucent. Add garlic and sauté until fragrant.
3. Add cauliflower rice and sauté for about 5-6 minutes. Remove from heat.
4. Sprinkle salt and pepper just before serving.

Ketogenic Snack Recipes

Healthy Granola Bars

Prep: 3 min	Total: 20 min	Servings: 15-20

Ingredients:

- 3 cups macadamia nuts
- 3 cups almonds
- 3 cups sunflower seeds
- 3 cups unsweetened flaked coconut
- 3 eggs
- 3/4 cup coconut butter
- 3/4 cup organic peanut butter
- 1 1/2 cups dark chocolate chips
- 3 tablespoons vanilla extract
- 3 teaspoons pumpkin pie spice

Method:

1. Blend together all the ingredients in a blender until nutty or smooth. If you like them nutty, then make a coarse paste. If you like it smooth, then blend for longer.
2. Transfer to a greased ovenproof dish. Press well.
3. Bake in a preheated oven at 350°F for 15 minutes or golden brown.
4. Cool slightly. Slice into pieces and serve.

Fish Fingers

Prep: 15 min	Total: 35 min	Servings: 6-8

Ingredients:

- 2 pounds' fish like cod or snapper, rinsed, cut into fingers
- 4 eggs, beaten
- 1 cup shredded coconut
- Sea salt to taste
- 1 teaspoon garlic powder
- 1/2 teaspoon pepper powder to taste
- 1/2 cup coconut oil

Method:

1. Add coconut, salt, garlic powder and pepper powder to a bowl.
2. First dip the fingers in the egg and then roll in the coconut mixture and set aside on a plate.
3. Add 1/4-cup oil to a skillet and place the skillet over medium heat.
4. Add some of the fingers and cook until brown.
5. Repeat step 3 and 4 with the remaining fingers.
6. Serve with any dip of your choice.

Fried Cheese Sticks

Prep: 10 min	Total: 30 min	Servings: 15

Ingredients:

- 15 cheese sticks, frozen (do not thaw)
- 2 eggs, beaten
- 4 tablespoons almond flour
- 2 tablespoons ground flax seeds
- 2 ounces' parmesan, grated
- 1 teaspoon baking powder
- 2 tablespoons water
- Oil as required (coconut oil or olive oil)

Method:

1. Place a small, deep frying pan over medium heat. Add oil. It should cover at least 2 inches from the bottom of the pan. Heat until the temperature of the oil is 375°F.
2. Meanwhile, mix together Parmesan, almond flour and baking powder in a bowl.
3. Add egg and water and beat well. Dip the frozen cheese sticks in this batter and immediately add to the hot oil. Cook until golden brown on all sides.
4. Remove with a slotted spoon and place onto paper towels.
5. Serve with a low-carb dip of your choice.

Pizza Bites

Prep: 15 min	Total: 35 min	Servings: 10-15

Ingredients:

For Pizza base:

- 3-ounce large pepperoni
- Pizza sauce, as much as required
- Grated cheese as required (optional)

For topping:

- Few olives, sliced
- 1 bell pepper, diced
- 3-4 mushrooms, chopped
- 1/2 cup green onions, chopped

Method:

1. Place the pepperoni slices on a lined baking sheet. Bake in a preheated oven at 400° F for about 7-8 minutes until the pepperoni is crisp.
2. Spread pizza sauce over each of the pepperoni. Sprinkle bell pepper, olives, mushrooms, green onions and cheese.
3. Bake for a few minutes until the cheese melts.

Ketogenic Dessert Recipes

Raspberry Chia Pudding

Prep: 5 min	Total: 19 min	Servings: 2

Ingredients:

- 1/2 cup vanilla flavored almond milk or soy milk, unsweetened
- 1/2 scoop vanilla protein powder
- 2 tablespoons raspberries, fresh or frozen
- 1 1/2 tablespoons chia seeds

Method:

1. Whisk together almond milk and protein powder.
2. Add chia seeds and mix well. Keep aside for 5-7 minutes. Stir again.
3. Repeat step 2.
4. Mix raspberries into it.
5. Keep aside for an hour in the refrigerator.

Berry Ice Cream

Prep: 10 min	Total: 4 hrs. 10 min	Servings: 6-8

Ingredients:

- 3 cups heavy whipping cream
- 1 1/2 cups blueberries or strawberries, or any other berries of your choice, unsweetened and extra for garnishing
- Few drops of stevia sweetener or any other sweetener of your choice (optional)

Method:

1. Add all the ingredients to a blender. Blend until smooth.
2. Freeze the ice cream for 5-6 hours or until set.
3. Remove from the freezer around 30 minutes before serving.
4. Garnish with the berries that you are using.

Strawberry Cheesecake

Prep: 10 min	Total: 2 hrs. 15 min	Servings: 6-8

Ingredients:

- 1 cup cream cheese, softened
- 1/2 cup heavy cream
- 4 eggs
- 2 teaspoons lemon juice
- 1 teaspoon vanilla extract
- Sugar substitute like stevia, to taste
- 1 cup frozen strawberries, thawed
- 1/2 cup strawberry slices
- Whipped cream to serve

Method:

1. Place cream cheese, heavy cream, eggs, lemon juice, vanilla extract, stevia and frozen strawberries in a microwave safe bowl. Whisk well until smooth.
2. Microwave on high for 90 seconds stirring in between.
3. Cool and refrigerate.
4. Serve chilled with fresh strawberry slices and whipped cream or any low-carb sauce.

Chocolate and Peanut Butter Bites

Prep: 15 min	Total: 4 hrs. 15 min	Servings: 8-10

Ingredients:

- 4 large Hass avocados, peeled, pitted, chopped
- 1/2 cup peanut butter, unsweetened
- 1/2 cup cocoa powder
- 20 drops liquid stevia or to taste (optional)

Method:

1. Blend together all the ingredients, except peanut butter, until smooth and creamy.
2. Pour into a freezer-safe container. Add peanut butter. With a knife, swirl the peanut butter.
3. Freeze until done.
4. Remove from the freezer 15 minutes before serving.
5. Scoop and serve.

Conclusion

To conclude, a lot of the "low-carb" diets are being pushed around, but most of them do not succeed for one crucial reason: they do not include consumption of high amounts of fat in the diet! Without a high amount of fat in the diet, you end up putting on weight and becoming extremely lethargic.

This is because without both carbohydrates and fats in your diet, your body has no source of energy. So, your body starts conserving the little protein you consume, breaking down some of it to power some of the more important bodily functions, while saving the bulk of it for future use, making you extremely lethargic. This also means that whatever fat you do consume goes into storage, resulting in weight gain.

This is why the Ketogenic Diet has seen a higher success rate over the bulk of low-carb diets. A little planning and you will be well on your way to losing those extra pounds without putting in a lot of effort!

I would like to take the opportunity to once again thank you for purchasing this book and I hope that you found the content of this book helpful!

Stay healthy; stay happy!

Vegan Ketogenic Diet

15-day Meal Plan

Free Gift Included

As part of our commitment to making sure you live a healthy lifestyle, we have included a free e-book in the link below. This book informs of the food groups and food items that will enable you to lose weight quickly. I hope that you enjoy this e-book and the extra gift as well. The link to the gift is below:

http://36potentfoodstoloseweightandlivehealthy.gr8.com

Disclaimer

About the Author

Sam Kuma is passionate about sharing his culinary experience with the world. His work involves the modernization of healthy diet plans. He has published many recipe books for vegan, ketogenic, Paleo diets and dash food cooking, along with several cookbooks on ethnic cuisines. His main focus is to make healthy diets like vegan and ketogenic mainstream by sharing easy-to-create and appetizing recipes. In his first two books regarding vegan recipes, he has produced delicious vegan chocolates, desserts, ice creams, burgers, and sandwiches. Below is a link to his other Amazon products:

Sam Kuma Special

Book Description

The Ketogenic diet is a fat based diet that aims at controlling the carbohydrate intake. It is a weight loss diet that is designed to help people shed excess weight. This book has been written to suit the needs of those who subscribe to the vegan diet and thus provides simple vegan ketogenic recipes.

The book also provides a 15-day ketogenic meal plan that will kick-start your diet. I am sure there are many books out there based on the Ketogenic diet but I am certain that none of them are as comprehensive and informative as this one.

The book is easy to navigate through and has been written for convenient reading. Here are some of the features of the book

- Simple recipes that can be prepared by just about anyone
- Recipes that use simple ingredients that are easily available
- A delectable breakfast menu
- A lunch and dinner menu designed to suit a wide palate
- Simple breakfast recipes
- A comprehensive 15-day meal plan to get you started

Once you get started with the diet, you will begin to experience a variety of changes both inside and outside your body. This book aims at helping you experience those changes and guide you through a permanent transformation.

So, what are you waiting for? Grab your copy today and get started.

Introduction

Firstly, I thank you for choosing this book and hope you have a good time reading it. Health is one of life's most important aspects. If you take your health for granted then you are bound to suffer the consequences. It, therefore, becomes important to focus on good health and eliminate unnecessary stress.

One good way of doing so is by following a strict diet. A diet can help you lose weight and maintain an ideal body. When we hear the word "diet" most of us assume we must deal with bland foods such as soups and stews. However, not all diets require you to settle for these types of foods; one such being the Ketogenic diet. The Ketogenic diet was originally designed to help epilepsy patients control their seizures but soon, doctors began to identify its positive impact on weight loss. They started to administer the diet to obese patients and noticed that they experienced positive results with it. Since then, the diet has been extensively used as a weight loss diet.

The Ketogenic diet promotes consumption of fats that are good for the body while reducing the carbohydrate intake. Carbohydrates are required by the body to carry out day-to-day activities. However, a modern diet is so high-carb that not all of it gets used up in a day. The spare gets stored in the body in the form of fat. This fat can sometimes turn into visceral fat, which is difficult to loosen and eliminate. The result will be an obese body that is incapable of burning the excessive fat deposits.

The Ketogenic diet aims at eliminating such a situation. It helps cut down on the carbohydrates that are converted to fat and promotes consumption of good fat that helps in breaking down the stored fat. There is widespread misconception that the Ketogenic is a meat-based diet. However, it can be modified to suit the tastes of both vegetarians and vegans.

The Vegan Ketogenic diet promotes consumption of fresh fruits, vegetables and whole grains that are free from chemical processing. It strictly forbids consumption of junk and processed foods that are capable of filling up the body with toxins. Apart from weight loss, the ketogenic diet provides a whole host of other benefits that are great for the body. Some of these include fighting illnesses such as cancer and cardiovascular disease, enhancing skin and hair health, increasing energy and building a strong immunity.

The diet is quite simple to adopt and anybody can take it up. You need not introduce a world of change in your existing diet to adopt the Ketogenic diet. You only have to make small changes to incorporate it.

Start by looking into your current diet and identifying the amount of carbohydrates you are taking in. Next, calculate exactly how much you need on a day-to-day basis. Come up with an exercise plan that can help you shed excess pounds while burning away the consumed carbohydrates.

To get you started on the meals to consume on the diet, this book provides simple ketogenic recipes that will give you a head start and push you on the right track. They have been tried and tested and designed to suit a wide palate. It also provides a 15-day meal plan that has been curated to suit the needs of those that wish to lose excess weight in little time.

I hope you use this book to experience positive results and change the way you look and feel about yourself.

Let us begin!

15 Day Meal Plan

Day 1

Breakfast - Keto Protein Pancakes

Lunch - Cream of Broccoli Soup

Snack - Keto Hummus

Dinner - Vegan Loaf

Desserts - Super Easy Keto Fudge

Day 2

Breakfast - Keto Breakfast Cereal

Lunch - Light Zucchini Soup

Snack - Cauliflower Popcorns

Dinner - Low Carb Pumpkin Cheddar Risotto

Desserts - Chocolate Pudding

Day 3

Breakfast - Breakfast Bowl

Lunch - Greek Salad

Snack - Parsnip Chips

Dinner - Tofu with Thai Coconut Peanut Sauce

Desserts - Strawberry Mousse

Day 4

Breakfast - Creamy Coconut Milk with Berries

Lunch - Tempeh Salad

Snack - Buffalo "Potato Wedges"

Dinner - Low Carb Pad Thai

Desserts - Vegan Keto Sugar Cookies

Day 5

Breakfast - Cheesecake Breakfast Bars

Lunch - Mushroom & Walnut Spicy Bolognese

Snack - Granola Bars

Dinner - Mock Tuna Salad

Desserts - Vegan Ketone Gingerbread Muffin's

Day 6

Breakfast - Tofu Scramble

Lunch - Courgette Rolls with Cauliflower and Broccoli Mash

Snack - Spicy Almonds

Dinner - Purple Cabbage & Pecan Salad

Desserts - No Bake Caramel Chocolate Slice

Day 7

Breakfast - Savory Indian Pancakes

Lunch - Eggplant Lasagna

Snack - Eggplant Fries

Dinner - Carrot and Zucchini Soup

Desserts - Mini Low Carb Peanut Butter Pumpkin Pie

Day 8

Breakfast - Coffee and Coconut Cup

Lunch - Creamy Tomato Soup without Cream

Snack - Smoked Zucchini Chips

Dinner - Mexican Cauliflower Rice

Desserts - Chocolate Chia Pudding

Day 9

Breakfast - Metabolism Boosting Hot Chocolate

Lunch - Jackfruit & Cauliflower Taco Bowls

Snack - Lettuce Wraps

Dinner - Chinese Hot and Sour Soup

Desserts - Vegan Keto Protein Brownies

Day 10

Breakfast - Green Smoothie

Lunch - Crispy Pressed Tofu with Garlic and Mint

Snack - Buffalo "Potato Wedges"

Dinner - Spicy Almond Tofu

Desserts - Nutty Blueberry Protein Balls

Day 11

Breakfast - Cherry Chocolate Protein Smoothie

Lunch - Collard Green Wraps

Snack - Cauliflower Popcorns

Dinner - Creamy Curry Noodle Bowl

Desserts - Chocolate Peanut Butter Low Carb Vegan Ice Cream

Day 12

Breakfast - Vanilla smoothie

Lunch - Shiritaki "Alfredo" with Spinach

Snack - Soy and Sesame Edamame

Dinner - Vegan Vegetable Moussaka

Desserts - Fresh Strawberry Lime Popsicles

Day 13

Breakfast - Green Goddess Smoothie

Lunch - Tempeh Lettuce Wraps

Snack - Lemon Poppy Tahini Salad Boats

Dinner - Cream of Mushroom Soup

Desserts - Vegan Keto Sugar Cookies

Day 14

Breakfast - Matcha Smoothie Bowl

Lunch - Cauliflower Chowder

Snack - Keto Hummus

Dinner - Vegan Fathead Pizza Crust

Desserts - Chocolate Pudding

Day 15

Breakfast - Cantaloupe Smoothie

Lunch - Vegan Keto Lo Mein

Snack - Granola Bars

Dinner - Vegan Cigkofte

Desserts - Vegan Ketone Gingerbread Muffin's

Chapter 1: Ketogenic Vegan Breakfast Recipes

Keto Protein Pancakes

Prep: 10 min	Total: 30 min	Servings: 8-12

Ingredients:

- 2 scoops plant based protein powder
- 4 tablespoons psyllium husk powder, soaked in a cup of water
- 2 tablespoons coconut oil
- 2 teaspoons baking powder
- ½ cup coconut flour
- 2 cups water
- 2 teaspoons vanilla extract

Instructions:

1. Add vanilla and coconut oil to the psyllium husk, which is soaked in water. Mix well and set aside for a while.
2. Mix together in a large bowl, protein powder, baking powder and coconut flour.
3. Add water and mix well.
4. Add the psyllium mixture into the bowl and mix until well combined.
5. Place a nonstick pan over medium heat. Pour about ¼ cup batter on it. Swirl the pan so that the batter spreads a little.
6. Cook until the underside is golden brown. Flip sides and cook the other side too.
7. Repeat the above 2 steps with the remaining batter.

Keto Breakfast Cereal

Prep: 15 min	Total: 17 min	Servings: 2

Ingredients:

- ¼ cup walnuts, chopped
- ¼ cup pecans, chopped
- 1/3 cups almonds, chopped
- ¼ cup blueberries
- 4 strawberries, chopped
- Sweetener (stevia or splenda) to taste (optional)
- Coconut milk or almond milk to serve

Instructions:

1. Mix together all the ingredients in a bowl. Divide into 2 bowls and serve with almond milk or coconut milk.

Breakfast Bowl

Prep: 10 min	Total: 12 min	Servings: 4

Ingredients:

- 2 medium avocadoes, peeled, pitted, halved
- 4 tablespoons tahini
- 1 large carrot, shredded

For dressing:

- 2 tablespoons lemon juice
- 2 tablespoons extra virgin olive oil
- ½ teaspoon ginger, grated
- ½ tablespoon poppy seeds
- 1/8 teaspoon salt

Instructions:

5. Whisk together all the ingredients of the dressing in a bowl. Set aside for a while for the flavors to set in.
6. Take ¼ cup of the dressing and add into a bowl. Add carrots to it. Mix well. You can use the remaining dressing over some salad.
7. Fill the avocado halves with it.
8. Top with tahini and serve.
9. Scoop along with the avocado and enjoy.

Creamy Coconut Milk with Berries

Prep: 2 min	Total: 3 min	Servings: 1

Ingredients:

- ½ cup berries (blackberries, raspberries or strawberries) fresh or frozen
- 2 ounce almonds
- 1 cup creamed coconut milk
- 1 large pinch cinnamon

Instructions:

1. Mix together all the ingredients in a bowl.
2. Serve. Tastes good when served cold.

Cheesecake Breakfast Bars

Prep: 5 min	Total: 30 min	Servings: 4

Ingredients:

- 2 ounces vegan cream cheese, softened
- ¼ cup canned coconut milk
- 1 scoop plant based vanilla protein powder
- ½ teaspoon ground cinnamon to sprinkle
- 1 tablespoon vegan butter, softened
- 2 tablespoons swerve or any other granulated sweetener
- 1 tablespoon coconut flour

Instructions:

1. Add cream cheese, butter and swerve into a bowl. Beat until creamy.
2. Add coconut milk and mix well. Add coconut flour and protein powder and mix well.
3. Transfer into a small greased baking dish. Sprinkle cinnamon over it.
4. Bake in a preheated oven at 350° F for about 20 minutes or until set.
5. Slice and serve.

Tofu Scramble

Prep: 20 min	Total: 30 min	Servings: 2-3

Ingredients:

- 16 ounces block extra firm tofu
- 1 red onion, thinly sliced
- 1 medium red bell pepper, finely chopped
- 4 cups kale, remove hard stems and ribs, roughly chopped
- 1 teaspoon cumin powder
- 2 tablespoons olive oil
- ½ teaspoon turmeric powder
- 1 teaspoon garlic powder
- ½ teaspoon chili powder
- 1 teaspoon sea salt or to taste
- 1 tablespoon fresh cilantro, chopped
- Low carb salsa to serve (optional)
- A dash of hot sauce

Instructions:

1. Place tofu over layers of paper towel. Place a heavy bottomed pan over it so that excess moisture is absorbed by the paper towel. Let it remain in this position for about 15- 20 minutes.
2. When done, remove the pan and crumble tofu into bite sized pieces.
3. Mix together in a small bowl all the dry spices and 2-3 tablespoons water and set aside.
4. Place a skillet over medium heat. Add oil and heat. Add onions and red pepper and cook until onions are translucent.

5. Add kale, salt and pepper. Mix well, cover and cook for about 2 minutes.
6. Push the vegetables to one side of the pan and add tofu to it. Sauté tofu for a couple of minutes and pour the spice mixture over tofu and vegetables and mix together tofu as well as the vegetables. Mix until well combined.
7. Cook for 6-7 minutes.
8. Add hot sauce and stir.
9. Garnish with cilantro and serve.

Savory Indian Pancakes

Prep: 15 min	Total: 35 min	Servings: 8

Ingredients:

- 2 cups full fat coconut milk
- 1 cup tapioca flour
- 1 cup almond flour
- 1 red onion, minced
- 2 Serrano pepper, minced
- ½ teaspoon turmeric powder
- ½ teaspoon Kashmiri chili powder
- 1 ½ teaspoons salt or to taste
- 1 inch pieces ginger, peeled, grated
- ¼ cup fresh cilantro leaves
- Pepper powder to taste
- Coconut oil or ghee or olive oil to make pancakes

Instructions:

1. Add almond flour, tapioca flour, turmeric powder, salt, pepper powder, and Kashmiri chili powder into a bowl.
2. Mix well and add coconut milk. Whisk until well combined.
3. Add onions, cilantro, Serrano pepper and ginger.
4. Place a nonstick pan over medium heat. Add about ½ teaspoon oil. Pour about a ladle full of batter into the pan. Swirl the pan to spread the batter. Cook until the underside is golden brown. Flip sides and cook the other side too.
5. Make pancakes with the remaining batter by following step 4.
6. Serve with mint or cilantro chutney.

120

Coffee and Coconut Cup

Prep: 5 min	Total: 7 min	Servings: 1

Ingredients:

- ¼ cup ground flaxseed,
- ¼ cup coconut flakes, unsweetened
- 2 tablespoons coconut oil
- 1 cup hot black coffee, unsweetened
- Liquid sweetener to taste

Instructions:

1. Add all the ingredients into a bowl. Whisk until well combined.
2. Pour into a mug and serve.

Metabolism Boosting Hot Chocolate

Prep: 3 min	Total: 10 min	Servings: 2

Ingredients:

- 2 scoops plant based chocolate protein powder
- ½ teaspoon ground cinnamon
- A pinch pepper powder
- ¼ cup canned coconut milk
- ¼ teaspoon cayenne pepper, chopped
- 2 cups water

Instructions:

1. Pour water into a saucepan and heat until it almost boils. Remove from heat.
2. Divide coconut milk and spices into 2 cups. Pour a little water into the cup and mix well.
3. Divide and add protein powder and pour the remaining water. Mix well and serve.

Green Smoothie

Prep: 8 min	Total: 10 min	Servings: 2

Ingredients:

- 4 cups spinach
- 2 cups coconut milk, chilled, unsweetened
- 4 Brazil nuts
- 2/3 cup almonds
- 2 tablespoons psyllium husk
- 2 scoops plant based protein powder
- 2 scoops greens powder
- 4 drops stevia or to taste (optional) or any other sweetener of your choice

Instructions:

5. Add spinach, almonds, Brazil nuts and coconut milk to a blender and blend until smooth.
6. Add rest of the ingredients and blend until smooth and creamy.
7. Pour into tall glasses.
8. Serve immediately with crushed ice.

Cherry Chocolate Protein Smoothie

Prep: 8 min	Total: 10 min	Servings: 2

Ingredients

- 2 cups coconut milk, unsweetened
- ¼ cup fresh cherries, pitted (If using frozen, thawed)
- 2/3 cup hemp hearts
- 2 scoops plant based protein powder
- ½ cup cocoa powder, unsweetened
- 1 teaspoon liquid chocolate stevia or to taste

Instructions:

1. Add all the ingredients to a blender and blend until smooth.
2. Pour into tall glasses and serve with crushed ice.

Vanilla smoothie

Prep: 5 min	Total: 7 min	Servings: 1

Ingredients:

- 1 tablespoon chia seeds or 1 tablespoon coconut butter
- ½ cup coconut milk
- 2 tablespoons plant based protein powder
- ½ tablespoon extra virgin coconut oil
- ½ teaspoon vanilla extract
- 3-4 drops stevia drops or to taste
- 3 tablespoons water

Instructions:

1. Add all the ingredients in a blender and blend until smooth.
2. Pour into a glass. Serve with crushed ice immediately.

Green Goddess Smoothie

Prep: 10 min	Total: 12 min	Servings: 2

Ingredients:

- 1 avocado, peeled, pitted, chopped
- 1 ¼ cups coconut milk
- ½ cup fresh baby spinach, rinsed
- ½ cup fresh mint leaves, rinsed
- 2 scoops plant based vanilla protein powder (or plain)
- ¼ cup pistachio nuts, unsalted
- 2 teaspoons vanilla extract
- 6 -10 drops liquid stevia
- 1 cup coconut water or plain water
- Few ice cubes

Instructions:

1   Add all the ingredients into a blender. Blend until smooth and creamy.
2   Transfer the smoothie into tall glasses.
3   Add crushed ice and serve.

Matcha Smoothie Bowl

Prep: 5 min	Total: 7 min	Servings: 2

Ingredients:

- 3 tablespoons goji berries
- 2 teaspoons matcha powder
- 2 tablespoons cacao nibs
- 3 tablespoons chia seeds
- 2 tablespoons coconut flakes
- 2 cups coconut yogurt
- 2 scoops greens powder (optional)

Instructions:

4. Add matcha powder, greens powder if using and yogurt into a blender and blend until smooth.
5. Pour into 2 individual serving bowls. Add cacao nibs, chia seeds and coconut flakes to it.
6. Stir, chill for a while and serve.

Berry Smoothie

Prep: 5 min	Total: 7 min	Servings: 2

Ingredients:

- 1 ¼ cups coconut milk, unsweetened
- 1 ½ cups almond milk, unsweetened
- ½ cup blueberries, fresh or frozen
- ½ cup raspberries, fresh or frozen
- ½ cup strawberries, fresh or frozen
- ½ cup walnuts
- Ice as required

Instructions:

1 Add strawberries, blueberries, raspberries, walnuts, coconut milk and almond milk to a blender.
2 Blend until the smoothie is smooth and creamy.
3 Transfer the smoothie into 2 tall glasses.
4 Add crushed ice and serve.

Cantaloupe Smoothie

Prep: 8 min	Total: 10 min	Servings: 1

Ingredients:

- 1 cup cantaloupe pieces
- ½ cup strawberries, chopped
- 4-5 romaine lettuce leaves

Instructions:

1. Add all the ingredients to the blender and blend until smooth. Add more water to dilute the smoothie if you desire a smoothie of thinner consistency.
2. Pour into tall glasses.
3. Serve with crushed ice.

Heart Healthy Smoothie

Prep: 10 min	Total: 12 min	Servings: 3

Ingredients:

- 2 cups red cabbage, chopped
- 2 Roma tomatoes
- 10 medium strawberries, chopped
- 1 red bell pepper, chopped
- 1 cup raspberries
- 2 cups cold water

Instructions:

1 Add all the ingredients to a blender and blend until smooth. Add more water to dilute the smoothie if you desire a smoothie of thinner consistency.
2 Pour in tall glasses.
3 Serve with ice.

Chapter 2: Ketogenic Vegan Soup Recipes

Cream of Broccoli Soup

Prep: 15 min	Total: 30 min	Servings: 6

Ingredients:

- 1 large cauliflower, broken into florets
- 6 cups broccoli, finely chopped
- 2 yellow onions, sliced
- 2 teaspoons extra virgin olive oil
- 5 cups almond milk, unsweetened
- 1 ½ teaspoons sea salt
- Freshly ground black pepper
- 2 tablespoons onion powder

Instructions:

5. Place a large saucepan over medium heat. Add oil. When the oil is heated, add onions and sauté until onions are translucent. Add salt, pepper, cauliflower and milk. Stir and bring to the boil.
6. Lower heat and cover with a lid. Simmer until soft. Add half the broccoli and remove from heat. Cool for a while.
7. Transfer into a blender and blend until smooth. Transfer it back into the saucepan.
8. Add remaining broccoli and onion powder and stir. Place the saucepan back on heat and simmer until broccoli is tender.
9. Ladle into soup bowls. Serve hot.

Light Zucchini Soup

Prep: 5 min	Total: 20 min	Servings: 2

Ingredients:

- 1 medium zucchini, chopped into cubes
- 2 cups vegetable stock
- 1 small onion, chopped
- 1 small chili pepper, chopped
- Salt to taste
- Pepper
- ¼ cup fresh dill, chopped
- 1 tablespoon olive oil

Instructions:

4. Place a pot over medium heat. Add oil. When the oil is heated, add onions and pepper. Sauté until onions are translucent.
5. Add stock, salt, and pepper. Simmer for 8-10 minutes. Add zucchini and simmer until tender. Remove from heat.
6. Add dill and serve either hot or cold. For cold, chill in the refrigerator.

Chilled Avocado Soup

Prep: 10 min	Total: 12 min	Servings: 4-5

Ingredients:

- 3 cups Hass avocado puree
- 3 cups vegetable broth
- 1 cup coconut cream (optional)
- ½ cup cilantro, chopped
- 2 jalapeno peppers, deseeded, chopped
- 2 teaspoons ground cumin
- 1 teaspoon salt or to taste

Instructions:

1. Add all the ingredients to a blender and blend until smooth.
2. Chill until use.
3. Serve in individual bowls.

Cream of Mushroom Soup

Prep: 10 min	Total: 40 min	Servings: 2

Ingredients:

- 3 cups cauliflower, chopped into florets
- 2 cups unsweetened almond milk
- 1 ½ teaspoons onion powder
- ½ teaspoon Himalayan rock salt
- Freshly ground pepper, to taste
- 1 teaspoon extra-virgin olive oil
- 2 ½ cups white mushrooms, sliced
- 1 yellow onion, chopped
- ½ teaspoon garlic powder

Instructions:

1. Place a saucepan over medium heat Add garlic, cauliflower, milk, onion powder, salt and pepper and stir. Bring to the boil.
2. Lower heat and cover with a lid. Simmer until the cauliflowers are soft. Remove from heat and puree the cauliflower using an immersion blender.
3. Meanwhile, place a saucepan over medium heat. Add oil. When the oil is heated, add onions and sauté for a couple of minutes. Add mushrooms and sauté until the onions are light brown.
4. Add the blended cauliflower. Mix well and bring to the boil.
5. Reduce heat and simmer for 10-12 minutes. If you find the soup too thick, add some more milk and heat thoroughly.
6. Ladle into individual soup bowls and serve hot.

Gazpacho

Prep: 15 min	Total: 25 min	Servings: 4

Ingredients:

- 4 ripe Roma tomatoes
- 1 small red onion, peeled, chopped
- 1 small cucumber, peeled, seeded, chopped
- ½ small green bell pepper, seeded, chopped
- ½ red pepper bell, seeded, chopped
- 2 large cloves garlic, peeled
- 1 red chili, seeded, stem removed
- Juice of half an orange
- 1 teaspoon orange zest, grated
- 1 tablespoon apple cider vinegar
- 6 tablespoons olive oil
- ½ cup tomato juice
- ½ cup cold water
- ½ teaspoon salt
- ¼ teaspoon pepper powder

For garnishing:

- 1 small cucumber, finely chopped
- 1 small red bell pepper, finely chopped
- 1 red onion, finely chopped

Instructions:

1. Place a saucepan over medium heat. Add tomatoes and bring to the boil. Boil until the skin just begins to crack. Remove from heat. Drain the water and pour cold water over it.
2. Peel the tomatoes, quarter and remove the seeds of the tomatoes.
3. Blend together tomatoes, peppers, cucumber, onion, chili, garlic, water, and orange zest in a blender until smooth.
4. Add olive oil, vinegar, orange juice, tomato juice, salt and pepper. Pulse for a few seconds. If you like it thinner in consistency, then add more tomato juice.
5. Refrigerate and serve chilled in bowls garnished with cucumber, red bell pepper and onions.

Carrot and Zucchini Soup

Prep: 15 min	Total: 55 min	Servings: 4

Ingredients:

- 2 large carrots, peeled, roughly chopped
- 1 apple, peeled, cored, roughly chopped
- 2 zucchinis, peeled, roughly chopped
- 1 tablespoon fresh ginger, minced
- ½ teaspoon turmeric
- 2 cups vegetable stock
- 1/ 8 teaspoon ground cinnamon
- Salt and pepper to taste
- 1 tablespoon coconut oil
- ½ cup coconut milk

Instructions:

1. Place a saucepan with oil over medium high heat. Add onions and sauté until translucent.
2. Add ginger and sauté for a couple of minutes. Add rest of the ingredients except coconut milk and bring to the boil.
3. Reduce heat and simmer for about 30 minutes. Blend with an immersion blender.
4. Add coconut milk, stir well and serve.

Cauliflower Chowder

Prep: 20 min	Total: 45 min	Servings: 10

Ingredients:

- 2 medium heads cauliflower, roughly chopped
- 2 large carrots, chopped
- 2 onions, diced
- 4 cloves garlic, minced
- 4 stalks celery, chopped
- 8 cups vegetable stock
- 2 cups coconut milk
- 1 tablespoon coconut oil
- 1 teaspoon ground coriander
- 1 teaspoon turmeric
- 1 ½ teaspoons ground cumin
- 2 tablespoons fresh dill, chopped
- Salt to taste
- Pepper to taste

Instructions:

1. Place a saucepan over medium high heat. Add oil. When the oil is heated, add onions, garlic, carrots and celery and sauté until onions are translucent.
2. Add cauliflower and sauté for about 5 minutes.
3. Add rest of the ingredients except dill and bring to the boil.
4. Lower heat and cover with a lid. Simmer until vegetables are tender.
5. Garnish with dill and serve.

Creamy Tomato Soup without Cream

Prep: 10 min	Total: 20 min	Servings: 4

Ingredients:

- 8 Roma tomatoes
- 1 cup sun dried tomatoes
- 1 cup raw macadamia nuts
- 2 teaspoons sea salt or to taste
- ½ cup fresh basil
- 1 teaspoon white pepper or to taste
- ¼ teaspoon black pepper
- 2 cloves garlic
- 4 cups water

Instructions:

1. Add all the ingredients into a blender and blend until smooth.
2. Transfer the contents to a large saucepan. Heat thoroughly.
3. Serve hot.

Chinese Hot and Sour Soup

Prep: 10 min	Total: 50 min	Servings: 3

Ingredients:

- 3 cups vegetable broth
- 1 cup mushrooms, sliced
- ½ small can bamboo shoots
- ½ small can water chestnuts
- 1 tablespoon soy sauce
- ¼ teaspoon pepper
- 1 teaspoon hot sauce
- 1 tablespoon vinegar
- 2 cloves garlic, minced
- ½ cup scallions sliced
- 1 tablespoon chili oil

Instructions:

1. Add all the ingredients except scallions and chili oil to a large pot. Place the pot over medium heat and bring to the boil.
2. Lower heat and cover with a lid. Simmer for about 20-25 minutes or until the vegetables are tender.
3. Add scallions and boil for 5 minutes. Taste and adjust the seasonings if required.
4. Ladle into soup bowls and serve.

Chapter 3: Ketogenic Vegan Salad Recipes

Greek Salad

Prep: 10 min	Total: 12 min	Servings: 4

Ingredients:

For salad:

- 2 cucumbers, chopped
- 8 tomatoes, chopped
- 1 red onion, thinly sliced
- 1 ½ cups Kalamata olives

For Greek style dressing:

- ¼ cup red wine vinegar
- ½ cup extra virgin olive oil
- 2 tablespoons fresh lemon juice
- 1 teaspoon dried oregano
- Sea salt to taste
- Freshly ground black pepper powder to taste

Instructions:

1. Add tomatoes, cucumber and red onions to a bowl and toss.
2. To make dressing: Add all the ingredients of the dressing into a bowl and whisk well.
3. Pour the dressing over the salad and toss well.
4. Top with olives and serve.

Cauliflower Salad

Prep: 10 min	Total: 40 min	Servings: 4

Ingredients:

- 2 cauliflowers, broken into florets
- 2 onions, sliced
- ¼ cup olive oil
- ½ cup baby spinach
- 1/3 cup sherry vinegar
- ½ cup fresh dill, snipped
- 1/3 cup almonds, toasted, slivered
- Salt to taste
- Pepper to taste

Instructions:

1. Add cauliflower to a baking dish. Sprinkle salt, pepper and olive oil. Toss well.
2. Roast in a preheated oven at 350° F for about 15 minutes.
3. Add onions, mix well and bake for another 15 minutes.
4. Meanwhile, make the dressing as follows: Whisk together vinegar, salt and pepper. Add almonds.
5. Add cauliflower to a bowl. Add spinach and dill. Pour dressing. Toss and serve.

Lemon Poppy Tahini Salad Boats

Prep: 10 min	Total: 15 min	Servings: 2

Ingredients:

- 7-8 lettuce leaves
- ½ cup sunflower seeds or tahini
- ½ cup purple cabbage, shredded

For dressing:

- 2 tablespoons lemon juice
- 2 tablespoons extra virgin olive oil
- ½ teaspoon ginger, grated
- ½ tablespoon poppy seeds
- 1/8 teaspoon salt
- Pepper to taste

Instructions:

1. Whisk together all the ingredients of the dressing in a bowl. Set aside for a while for the flavors to set in.
2. Mix together in a bowl, cabbage, sunflower seeds and dressing.
3. Place lettuce leaves on a serving platter. Place the cabbage mixture on the lettuce leaves and serve.

Cauliflower Tabbouleh

Prep: 15 min	Total: 16 min	Servings: 4

Ingredients:

- 4 cups cauliflower, grated or finely chopped
- ¼ cup fresh mint leaves, chopped
- 1 cup fresh parsley, chopped
- 2 cups fresh tomatoes, chopped
- ¼ cup lemon juice
- Pepper to taste
- Salt to taste
- ½ cup olive oil
- 2 tablespoons lemon zest

Instructions:

1. Add all the ingredients in a bowl and toss until well combined.
2. Chill for an hour.
3. Mix well and serve.

Tempeh Salad

Prep: 20 min	Total: 22 min	Servings: 4

Ingredients:

- 2 cups tempeh, cubed
- 2 sticks celery, chopped
- 1 onion, chopped
- 2 medium pickles, chopped
- ¼ cup parsley, minced
- 1 ½ tablespoons soy sauce
- 2 tablespoons curry powder or to taste
- 2 cloves garlic minced
- 2 tablespoons mustard

Instructions:

1. Steam the tempeh. Cool completely.
2. Add all the ingredients to a large bowl. Toss well, chill for a couple of hours and serve.

Mock Tuna Salad

Prep: 15 min	Total: 16 min	Servings: 8

Ingredients:

- 2 cups extra firm tofu, drained, pressed, cubed
- ½ cup carrots, finely chopped
- ½ cup celery, finely chopped
- 1 teaspoon kelp powder
- 2 teaspoons lemon juice
- 1 cup vegan mayonnaise
- 2 teaspoons onion powder
- Salt to taste
- Pepper to taste
- Seaweed snacks to serve
- Celery sticks to serve

Instructions:

1. Add all the ingredients into a bowl and toss well.
2. Top with celery sticks and seaweed snacks and serve.

Thai Salad

Prep: 15 min	Total: 17 min	Servings: 2

Ingredients:

- ½ cup carrots, peeled, chopped
- ¼ cup cilantro, chopped
- 1 clove garlic, minced
- Juice of ½ a lemon
- 1 ½ cups kale, chopped
- 1 cup Napa cabbage, chopped
- 1 red bell pepper, chopped
- 1 cup thin coconut milk
- 2 tablespoons creamy peanut butter
- ½ teaspoon Sriracha sauce
- ½ teaspoon yellow curry powder
- Kosher salt to taste

Instructions:

3. To make the dressing: Add garlic, lemon juice, peanut butter, curry powder, and coconut milk to a bowl and whisk well.
4. Mix together rest of the ingredients in a large bowl. Add the dressing and toss well.
5. Serve.

Purple Cabbage & Pecan Salad

Prep: 10 min	Total: 12 min	Servings: 4

Ingredients:

For the salad:

- 8 cups purple cabbage, thinly sliced
- ½ cup Chinese pecans
- 2 scallions, chopped, green as well as the white parts

For the dressing:

- ¼ cup vinegar
- ¼ cup sugar
- 2 tablespoons olive oil
- 2 tablespoons soy sauce

Instructions:

1. Mix together in a bowl, all the ingredients of the dressing.
2. Mix together in a large bowl the rest of the ingredients.
3. Pour the dressing over the salad and toss.
4. Serve immediately.

Chapter 4: Ketogenic Vegan Snacks / Appetizer Recipes

Keto Hummus

Prep: 10 min	Total: 12 min	Servings: 12

Ingredients:

- 2 cups zucchini, peeled, chopped
- ¼ cup fresh lemon juice
- 2 cloves garlic, peeled
- ½ tablespoon ground cumin
- 6 tablespoons tahini
- 2 tablespoons olive oil
- 1 teaspoon salt or to taste

To garnish:

- 2 tablespoons fresh parsley, chopped
- 1 tablespoon olive oil
- ¼ teaspoon paprika

Instructions:

1. Add all the ingredients into a blender and blend until smooth. Transfer into a bowl.
2. Garnish with parsley and paprika. Drizzle olive oil on top and serve.
3. A serving is of 2 tablespoons.

Cauliflower Popcorns

Prep: 10 min	Total: 1 hr. 10 min	Servings: 8

Ingredients:

- 2 heads cauliflower, chopped into small florets (about an inch)
- ½ cup olive oil
- Salt to taste
- ½ teaspoon red pepper flakes

Instructions:

1. Add olive oil and salt to a large bowl. Whisk well.
2. Add cauliflower florets and toss until well combined.
3. Line a large baking sheet with parchment paper. Transfer the cauliflower on to the baking sheet. Spread it all over the sheet.
4. Bake in a preheated oven at 375° F for about an hour or until the cauliflower is golden brown.

Parsnip Chips

Prep: 10 min	Total: 20 min	Servings: 6

Ingredients:

- 3 medium parsnips, cut into ¼ inch thick round slices
- 3 tablespoons extra virgin olive oil
- Garlic powder (optional)
- ¼ teaspoon salt or to taste
- ¼ black pepper powder
- ½ teaspoon paprika
- Any dried herbs of your choice like rosemary or dill (optional)

Instructions:

1. Brush the parsnip slices on both sides with olive oil. Place the parsnip slices on a lined baking sheet.
2. Sprinkle salt, pepper, paprika and herbs, garlic powder if you are using
3. Lay the parsnip slices in a single layer.
4. Bake in a preheated oven at 400° F for 10 minutes or until crisp. Turn the chips once half way through baking.
5. Remove from the oven. Cool on a wire rack and serve.

Note: You can make chips with kale or zucchinis or sweet potatoes in a similar manner.

Only the baking time varies.

Granola Bars

Prep: 15 min	Total: 20 min	Servings: 12

Ingredients:

- 1½ cups mixed nuts and seeds of your choice
- ½ cup dried cranberries
- 1 cup unsweetened, shredded coconut
- 2 tablespoons coconut oil
- ¼ cup sunflower seed butter
- Swerve sweetener or stevia to taste
- ¼ teaspoon vanilla extract
- ¼ teaspoon sea salt
- ½ teaspoon ground cinnamon

Instructions:

1. Line a Pyrex dish with parchment paper and set aside.
2. Chop half the nuts into small pieces. Add rest of the nuts to the food processor and pulse until the pieces are smaller than the chopped pieces.
3. Add all the nuts to a bowl. Add cranberries and shredded coconut and mix well.
4. Add coconut oil, sunflower butter, honey, vanilla, salt and cinnamon to a small saucepan. Place the saucepan over medium–low heat. When it starts bubbling, remove from heat.
5. Pour this mixture into the bowl of nuts and stir well. Transfer the entire contents into the prepared dish. Spread all over the dish. Press well and keep aside for 2 hours.
6. Cover and place in the freezer for an hour.

7. Slice into bars and serve.

Spicy Almonds

Prep: 5 min	Total: 35 min	Servings: 12

Ingredients:

- 3 cups almonds
- 1 tablespoon extra-virgin olive oil
- 1 ½ teaspoon ground cumin
- 1 ½ teaspoons ground coriander
- 1 teaspoon chili powder
- 1 ½ teaspoons curry powder (optional)
- ½ teaspoon sea salt
- ¼ teaspoon cayenne pepper or to taste

Instructions:

1. Place the almonds in a baking dish. Add rest of the ingredients into the dish and toss well.
2. Bake in a preheated oven at 350° F for about 30 minutes or until done.
3. Cool and store in an airtight container

Note: Almonds can be replaced with macadamia nuts or any nuts of your choice.

Eggplant Fries

Prep: 10 min	Total: 30 min	Servings: 6-8

Ingredients:

- 2 medium eggplants, chopped into 1 cm rounds and then cut into 1 cm strips
- 2 tablespoons olive oil
- Salt to taste
- Pepper powder to taste
- Garlic powder to taste

Instructions:

1. Place the eggplant strips on a baking sheet. Brush with oil.
2. Sprinkle salt, garlic powder, and pepper.
3. Bake in a preheated oven at 400° F for about 20 minutes or until brown,
4. Sprinkle more salt, garlic powder, and pepper and serve.

Smoked Zucchini Chips

Prep: 10 min	Total: 55 min	Servings: 4-6

Ingredients:

- 3 medium zucchinis
- Salt to taste
- 2 tablespoons olive oil
- 3 teaspoons smoked paprika or to taste
- Pepper powder to taste

Instructions:

1. Cut the zucchini into ¼ inch thick slices, crosswise with a slicer or a knife.
2. Place the zucchini on a sieve in layers, sprinkled with salt and pepper for the moisture to drain out.
3. Pat dry the zucchini slices with a paper towel and place on a greased baking tray.
4. Brush the top of the zucchini slices with oil. Sprinkle paprika and pepper.
5. Bake in a preheated oven at 250° F for 45 minutes. Turn off the oven and let the chips remain inside for an hour so that it remains crispy.
6. Transfer into airtight container when cooled.

Lettuce Wraps

Prep: 10 min	Total: 13 min	Servings: 8

Ingredients:

- 8 leaves iceberg lettuce
- 1 large carrot, cut into matchsticks
- ½ cucumber, cut into matchsticks
- ½ cup keto hummus
- ¼ teaspoon paprika

Instructions:

1. Spread lettuce leaves on your working area.
2. Divide and place carrots and cucumber over the leaves. Add a tablespoon of hummus. Sprinkle paprika.
3. Roll and serve.

Buffalo "Potato Wedges"

Prep: 10 min	Total: 55 min	Servings: 4-6

Ingredients:

- 4 medium rutabagas, rinsed, peeled, chopped into wedges
- 1 cup vegan buffalo wings sauce
- 8 tablespoons vegan butter, melted
- 1 teaspoon onion powder
- 4 green onions, chopped
- 1 teaspoon salt or taste
- Pepper powder to taste

Instructions:

1. Add butter, salt, onion powder and black pepper powder to a bowl. Dip rutabaga wedges and coat it well.
2. Place the wedges on a lined baking sheet in one layer.
3. Bake in a preheated oven at 400° F for about 30 minutes.
4. Remove from oven and pour Buffalo wings sauce, toss and bake for another 15 minutes.
5. Remove from the oven, serve garnished with green onions.

Soy and Sesame Edamame

Prep: 1 min	Total: 5 min	Servings: 4

Ingredients:

- 3 cups edamame in pods
- 2 teaspoons soy sauce
- Pepper to taste
- Salt to taste
- 4 tablespoons sesame oil, toasted

Instructions:

1. Place a pot of water over medium heat. Bring to the boil. Add edamame and boil for 5 minutes.
2. Drain and add into a bowl of cold water. Drain and pat dry.
3. Place a pan over high heat. Add sesame oil. When the oil is well heated, add edamame and sauté until light brown.
4. Add soy sauce and cook until dry.
5. Add salt and a generous sprinkle of pepper. Mix well.
6. Serve either hot or chilled.

Chapter 5: Ketogenic Vegan Main Course Recipes

Cauliflower Rice

Prep: 10 min	Total: 20 min	Servings: 4

Ingredients:

- 2 heads cauliflower, chopped into florets
- 1 onion, finely diced
- 4 tablespoons olive oil
- 4 cloves garlic, minced
- Salt to taste
- Pepper powder to taste

Instructions:

5. Add the cauliflower florets to the food processor bowl and pulse until you get rice like texture. Alternately, grate the cauliflower.
6. Place a large nonstick skillet over medium high heat. Add oil. When the oil is heated, add onions and sauté until translucent. Add garlic and sauté for about a minute until fragrant.
7. Add cauliflower rice and sauté for about 5-6 minutes. Remove from heat.
8. Sprinkle salt and pepper just before serving.
9. Serve hot with a sauce or curry of your choice.

Mexican Cauliflower Rice

Prep: 15 min	Total: 30 min	Servings: 6

Ingredients:

- 6 cups cauliflower florets
- 1 large onion, chopped
- 2 jalapeños, finely chopped + extra to garnish
- 1 ½ cups bell pepper, diced
- 8 cloves garlic, minced
- 4 medium tomatoes, finely chopped
- 2 teaspoons ground cumin
- Salt to taste
- 1 teaspoon paprika or chili powder
- 2 tablespoons lime juice
- 1 avocado, peeled, pitted, sliced
- 2 tablespoons olive oil
- 2 tablespoons fresh cilantro, chopped

Instructions:

1. Add the cauliflower florets to the food processor bowl and pulse until you get rice like texture. Alternately, grate the cauliflower.
2. Place a large nonstick skillet over medium high heat. Add oil. When the oil is heated, add onions and sauté until translucent. Add garlic and jalapeños and sauté for about a minute until fragrant.
3. Add tomatoes, cumin, paprika and salt and sauté until tomatoes are soft.

4. Add cauliflower rice and bell pepper and sauté for about 5-6 minutes. Remove from heat.
5. Divide and serve in plates. Garnish with cilantro. Drizzle lemon juice. Place avocado slices over it and serve.

Tempeh Lettuce Wraps

Prep: 10 min	Total: 18 min	Servings: 8

Ingredients:

- 2 packages tempeh, crumbled
- 1 onion, chopped
- 1 red bell pepper, chopped
- 2 heads butter leaf lettuce - 8 leaves
- 2 tablespoons olive oil
- 2 tablespoons garlic, chopped
- 2 tablespoons low sodium soy sauce
- 2 teaspoons garlic powder
- 2 teaspoons ginger powder
- 2 teaspoons onion powder
- Salt to taste

Instructions:

1. Place a large pan over medium heat. Add oil. When the oil is heated, add garlic and sauté until fragrant.
2. Add onions, tempeh and bell pepper and sauté until onions are translucent.
3. Add soy sauce, garlic powder, ginger powder, onion powder and salt and cook for a couple of minutes.
4. Spread the lettuce leaves on your work area. Spread the tempeh mixture over the leaves. Roll and serve.

Jackfruit & Cauliflower Taco Bowls

Prep: 12 min	Total: 22 min	Servings: 6

Ingredients:

- 2 cans young jackfruit in water, drained, chopped into smaller pieces
- 2 cups frozen kale
- 1 teaspoon onion powder to taste
- 1 teaspoon garlic powder or to taste
- 2 tablespoons olive oil
- 2 tablespoons taco seasoning or chili powder or to taste
- 8 cups cauliflower florets

To serve:

- Guacamole
- Vegan cheese

Instructions:

1. Add the cauliflower florets to the food processor bowl and pulse until you get rice like texture. Alternately, grate the cauliflower.
2. Place a large nonstick skillet over medium high heat. Add oil. When the oil is heated, add onions and sauté until translucent. Add garlic and sauté for about a minute until fragrant.
3. Add cauliflower rice and sauté for about 5-6 minutes. Remove from heat.
4. Divide and serve in bowls. Top with guacamole and vegan cheese and serve.

Crispy Pressed Tofu with Garlic and Mint

Prep: 15 min	Total: 27 min	Servings: 2

Ingredients:

- 14 ounce package extra firm tofu
- 2 tablespoons extra virgin olive oil
- ¼ cup fresh mint leaves, chopped
- Zest of ½ lemon, finely grated
- 2 large cloves garlic
- ¾ teaspoon sea salt or to taste
- 2 tablespoons lemon juice
- ½ teaspoon red pepper flakes or to taste

Instructions:

1. Slice tofu into 2 thick slices. Place on layers of paper towel and press to remove excess moisture.
2. Mix together rest of the ingredients in a bowl.
3. Add tofu and mix well. Let the tofu marinate for a minimum of 30 minutes.
4. Place a nonstick pan over medium heat. Remove the tofu from the marinade and place on the pan. Cook until the underside is golden brown. Flip sides and cook the other side until golden brown.
5. Remove and place on a serving platter.
6. Pour the marinade into the pan and cook for a couple of minutes.
7. Pour over the cooked tofu and serve immediately.

Collard Green Wraps

Prep: 10 min	Total: 20 min	Servings: 6 -8

Ingredients:

- 4 cups walnuts
- 3 teaspoons chili powder or to taste
- 14 teaspoon cayenne pepper
- 2 tablespoons ground cumin
- 3 teaspoons ground coriander
- 12 large collard green leaves, discard stems, trimmed 2 inches from the bottom of the leaves
- 4 tablespoons low sodium tamari
- Salsa as required

Instructions:

1. Add walnuts into the food processor bowl and pulse until the walnuts are coarse in texture. Transfer into a bowl and add the spices and tamari and mix well.
2. Spread the collard leaves with the light side facing up on your work area.
3. Divide the mixture among the leaves. Spoon about a tablespoon of salsa over it. Fold the sides over the filling and roll tightly.
4. Cut into 2 and serve with some more salsa.

Cauliflower and Pumpkin Dal

Prep: 15 min	Total: 45 min	Servings: 4

Ingredients:

- 1 pound pumpkin or butternut squash, peeled, chopped into small pieces
- 1 medium onion, finely chopped
- 1 small head cauliflower, chopped into small florets
- 1 ½ tablespoons coconut oil
- 2 cloves garlic, minced
- ½ tablespoon ginger, grated
- ½ teaspoon cumin powder
- ½ teaspoon turmeric powder
- ¼ teaspoon red chili flakes
- 1 teaspoon mild curry powder
- 1 cup vegetable stock
- 1 tablespoon lime juice
- ½ cup coconut cream + extra for garnishing
- 2 tablespoons sesame seeds + extra for garnishing
- 2 tablespoons fresh cilantro, chopped
- ½ teaspoon salt or to taste

Instructions:

1. Place a large skillet over medium heat. Add coconut oil. When the oil melts, add onions and sauté until onions are light golden brown.
2. Add pumpkin, ginger and garlic. Sauté for a couple of minutes until fragrant.

3. Add turmeric, cumin, curry powder and chili flakes and sauté for a few seconds.
4. Add vegetable stock, coconut cream, lime juice, salt and sesame seeds. Mix well and bring to a boil.
5. Lower heat and cover with a lid. Simmer for about 10 minutes.
6. Meanwhile place the cauliflower in the food processor bowl and process until it is of fine texture or make it of rice like texture.
7. Add cauliflower. Stir, cover and cook until done. Mash with a potato masher.
8. Garnish with cilantro, sesame seeds and coconut cream.

Creamy Curry Noodle Bowl

Prep: 15 min	Total: 25 min	Servings: 8

Ingredients:

- 2 full packets kanten noodles
- 1 head cauliflower, chopped
- 4 carrots, julienned
- 2 red bell pepper, chopped
- 8 cups mixed greens
- ½ cup fresh cilantro, chopped

For creamy curry sauce:

- ½ cup tahini or avocado oil mayonnaise
- ½ cup water

- 4 teaspoons curry powder
- 1 teaspoon ground turmeric
- 3 teaspoons ground coriander
- 2 teaspoons ground cumin
- ½ teaspoon ground ginger
- 1 teaspoon black pepper
- 2 teaspoons sea salt or to taste
- 4 tablespoons avocado oil or MCT oil
- 4 tablespoons apple cider vinegar

Instructions:

1. To make curry sauce: Add all the ingredients of the curry sauce into a blender and blend until smooth. Set aside.
2. Place the noodles sheets in a large bowl and pour hot water over it (not boiling hot but more than warm). Soak for about 5 minutes. Drain and set aside.
3. Add cauliflower, carrots, bell peppers, and cilantro and mix well.
4. Place salad greens on individual serving plates. Place the noodles and vegetables over it.
5. Pour creamy curry sauce over it and serve. It can be chilled and served later too.

Eggplant Lasagna

Prep: 20 min	Total: 1 hr. 30 min	Servings: 8

Ingredients:

- 3 pounds eggplants, sliced into 2 mm rounds
- 2 cups vegan mozzarella cheese, sliced
- 4 cans (15 ounces each) diced tomatoes, unsalted
- 2 pounds mushrooms, sliced
- 2 large onions, diced
- 5-6 cloves garlic, minced
- 2 tablespoons olive oil
- 3-4 tablespoons Italian seasoning
- Salt to taste
- Pepper to taste
- Cooking spray

Instructions:

1. To make sauce: Place a large skillet with oil over medium high heat. Add garlic and sauté for about a minute until fragrant.
2. Add onions and sauté until translucent. Add mushrooms and cook until brown. Add rest of the ingredients except eggplant and cheese. Mix well and bring to the boil.
3. Reduce heat and cover with a lid. Simmer for 8-10 minutes. Stir once in a while. Uncover and cook for another 15 minutes stirring occasionally.
4. Line a large rectangular baking dish with aluminum foil. Spray with cooking spray. Place half the eggplants in a single layer without overlapping. Spread half the sauce over it.
5. Place the remaining eggplant slices over the sauce. Spread the remaining sauce over it. Cover with foil.
6. Bake in a preheated oven at 325° F for 30 minutes. Raise the temperature to 375° F and bake for another 30 minutes.

7. Remove from the oven. Remove the foil and place the cheese slices all over the dish. Bake until cheese is melted. Let it remain in the oven for 10 minutes before serving.

Vegan Loaf

Prep: 15 min	Total: 1 hr. 15 min	Servings: 8

Ingredients:

- 2 cups mushrooms, chopped
- 1 red onion, diced
- 2 tablespoons coconut oil
- 1 cup sunflower seeds
- 1 cup finely ground almond flour
- ½ teaspoon Himalayan rock salt
- 4 cloves garlic, minced
- 2 tablespoons finely ground flaxseed
- 6 tablespoons warm water
- 2 cups hemp hearts
- 4 teaspoons spice mixture of your choice

Instructions:

1. Grease 2 medium size loaf pans with oil and set aside.
2. Add onions, garlic and mushrooms and sauté until light brown. Remove from heat and set aside.
3. Mix together ground flaxseed with 6 tablespoons water and set aside for 5 minutes.
4. Add sunflower seeds to the food processor bowl. Pulse until they become smaller in size. Add hemp hearts, almond flour, spice mixture and salt. Pulse until well combined and hem hearts are smaller in size.

5. Transfer into a bowl. Add the sautéed onion mixture into the food processor bowl and pulse until they are small bits. Transfer into the bowl of hemp heart mixture.
6. Mix well. Add the flaxseed mixture and mix well. Divide the mixture into 2 parts and place each in the prepared loaf pans.
7. Bake in a preheated oven at 350° F for 40-45 minute or until a toothpick when inserted in the center comes out clean.
8. Remove from the oven and cool for a couple of hours. Run a knife around the edges of the bread and remove the loaf. Slice and serve.

Low Carb Pumpkin Cheddar Risotto

Prep: 15 min	Total: 35 min	Servings: 6

Ingredients:

- 1 small onion, chopped
- 6 cups cauliflower, made into rice
- 6 ounces vegan cheddar cheese, shredded
- 4 tablespoons vegan butter
- Pepper to taste
- Salt to taste
- 1cup pumpkin or butternut squash puree
- 4 teaspoons paprika or to taste
- ½ cup dry white wine (optional)

Instructions:

1. Place a large saucepan over medium heat. Add vegan butter and melt. Add onion and sauté until translucent. Add paprika, salt and pepper and stir for a few seconds.
2. Add wine if using and stir. Add pumpkin puree and cauliflower and mix well.
3. Cover with a lid and simmer for 15 minutes or until the cauliflower turns soft. Stir a couple of times while it is cooking. Taste and adjust the seasoning if necessary.
4. Remove from heat. Add vegan cheddar cheese and stir.
5. Serve hot.

Easy Carrot Slaw with Smoky Maple Tempeh Triangles

Prep: 15min	Total: 20 min	Servings: 8

Ingredients:

- 16 ounces tempeh, sliced into triangles
- 5-6 teaspoons tamari or soy sauce
- 8 cups carrots, shredded
- 2 tablespoons walnuts, crushed
- 2 small onions, diced
- ½ teaspoon liquid smoke (optional)
- 2 teaspoons extra virgin olive oil or virgin coconut oil
- 2 tablespoons curry powder
- ¼ teaspoon pepper powder or to taste
- ½ teaspoon ground turmeric
- 4 tablespoons tahini
- 1 cup flat leaf parsley, finely chopped, + extra to garnish
- ½ cup lemon juice
- ½ teaspoon cayenne pepper or to taste
- Salt to taste

Instructions:

1. Place a skillet over high heat. Add oil. When the oil is heated, add tempeh, tamari and liquid smoke.
2. Cook until all the liquid is absorbed and the edges are browned. Flip the tempeh frequently while it is cooking.
3. Add walnut and pepper and mix well. Remove from heat and cover. Set aside for a while.

4. Mix together rest of the ingredients into a bowl and divide into individual serving plates. Place tempeh on top and serve.

Shiritaki "Alfredo" with Spinach

Prep: 5 min	Total: 13 min	Servings: 4

Ingredients:

- 2 packages shiritaki noodles, drained, rinsed
- 2 cups frozen spinach
- 4 ounces vegan cream cheese
- Salt to taste
- Pepper to taste
- ½ teaspoon garlic powder
- 2 tablespoons olive oil
- Almond milk as required

Instructions:

1. Add all the ingredients into a skillet. Place the skillet over medium heat. Add almond milk as required and stir. Heat thoroughly.
2. Transfer into bowls and serve.

Vegan Keto Lo Mein

Prep: 10 min	Total: 20 min	Servings: 4

Ingredients:

- 2 packages kelp noodles
- 2 cups frozen spinach
- 1 cup shelled edamame
- ½ cup carrots, julienned
- ½ cup mushrooms, sliced

For the sauce:

- 4 tablespoons tamari or soy sauce
- 1 teaspoon ground ginger
- ½ teaspoon Sriracha sauce
- 2 tablespoons sesame oil
- 1 teaspoon garlic powder

Instructions:

1. Soak the kelp noodles in a bowl of water for a while. Drain and set aside.
2. To make sauce: Place a saucepan over medium low heat. Add all the ingredients of the sauce into the saucepan and heat.
3. When the sauce is heated, add noodles and mix well. Add some water if desired so that the mixture is not very dry.
4. Cook until the noodles are soft. Remove from heat.
5. Divide and serve in bowls.

Spicy Almond Tofu

Prep: 10 min	Total: 30 min	Servings: 4

Ingredients:

- 2 packages firm tofu or extra firm tofu
- 4 tablespoons soy sauce
- 4 tablespoons water
- ½ teaspoon onion powder
- ½ teaspoon garlic powder
- ½ teaspoon paprika
- Salt to taste
- Pepper to taste
- ½ teaspoon chili flakes
- 2 tablespoons sesame seeds, divided
- 2 teaspoons sesame oil
- 2 tablespoons coconut oil
- 4 tablespoons green chili sauce
- ¼ cup almonds, sliced
- Steamed broccoli to serve

Instructions:

1. Place tofu on paper towels. Place a heavy skillet over the tofu to drain out excess moisture. Chop into cubes.
2. Place a skillet over high heat. Add coconut oil. When the oil is heated, add tofu and sauté until golden brown.

3. Add almonds and cook for a couple of minutes. Add rest of the ingredients except ½ tablespoon sesame seeds and sesame seeds and cook until dry.
4. Place steamed broccoli in bowls. Place tofu on top. Drizzle sesame oil over it. Sprinkle remaining sesame seeds on top and serve.

Low Carb Pad Thai

Prep: 10 min	Total: 13 min	Servings: 2

Ingredients:

- ½ bag kelp noodles
- 1 small white onion
- 2 cloves garlic, peeled
- 4 tablespoons natural peanut butter
- 2 tablespoons soy sauce or tamari or liquid aminos
- 1 teaspoon red pepper flakes
- 2 tablespoons lime juice
- 1 tablespoon sesame seeds, toasted
- 2 tablespoons scallions, chopped
- 2 tablespoons cilantro, chopped
- Salt to taste
- Pepper powder to taste

Instructions:

1. Add kelp noodles to a bowl of water and soak for a while.
2. Add peanut butter, onion, tamari, lime juice, garlic, pepper flakes, pepper, and salt into a blender and blend until smooth and creamy.
3. Drain the noodles and place in a large bowl. Pour the peanut butter mixture over it and toss well.
4. Sprinkle sesame seeds, scallions, and cilantro and serve.

Vegan Fathead Pizza Crust

Prep: 5 min	Total: 35 min	Servings: 4

Ingredients:

- 1 cup whole flaxseeds, finely ground
- 4 tablespoons psyllium powder
- ½ cup vegan cream cheese
- 2 teaspoons baking powder
- 2 teaspoons garlic powder
- 1 teaspoon salt or to taste
- 1 cup water

For topping:

- Pizza sauce or pesto (keto friendly)
- Vegan cheese as required
- Vegetables of your choice, sliced

Instructions:

1. Add all the dry ingredients into a bowl and mix well. Add vegan cream cheese and mix well.
2. Add water, a little at a time and mix well to form dough.
3. Divide the dough into 2 and shape into 2 balls. Place on a baking sheet. Flatten to shape into a pizza.
9. Bake in a preheated oven at 350° F for about 25 minutes. Flip sides and bake for 5 more minutes
4. Remove from the oven and spread sauce over it. Top with vegetables and finally vegan cheese.
5. Place it back in the oven. Bake for about 10-15 minutes.
6. Chop into wedges and serve.

Ultimate Keto Falafel

Prep: 15 min	Total: 45 min	Servings: 5

Ingredients:

- 1 cup hemp hearts
- 2 tablespoons fresh parsley, chopped
- 1 small onion, chopped
- 2 tablespoons fresh cilantro, chopped
- 1 teaspoon ground cumin
- 2 teaspoons flax meal mixed with 4 teaspoons water
- 2 teaspoons baking powder
- 4 cloves garlic
- Salt to taste
- Coconut oil or olive oil to fry

To serve:

- 5 cups lettuce, sliced
- 1 small cucumber, thinly sliced
- 1 tomato, thinly sliced

Instructions:

1. Add all the ingredients except flaxseed mixture into the food processor and pulse until well combined.
2. Add flaxseed mixture and pulse again. Divide the mixture into 10 equal portions. Shape each into falafels.
3. Place a nonstick pan over medium heat. Add about a tablespoon of oil. When the oil is heated, place the falafels on it (cook in batches).

4. Cook until the underside is golden brown. Flip sides and cook the other side until golden brown.
5. Place a cup of lettuce on 5 serving plates. Place 2 falafels on each plate. Top with slices of tomato and cucumber. Serve with keto hummus.

Courgette Rolls with Cauliflower and Broccoli Mash

Prep: 20 min	Total: 55 min	Servings: 5

Ingredients:

- 3 big courgettes
- 2 onions, finely chopped
- 1 block vegan cheese
- 2 peppers, finely chopped
- 8 cloves garlic, finely chopped + extra to top
- 2 tablespoons pesto
- Salt to taste
- Pepper to taste
- 1 tablespoon olive oil + extra to drizzle
- 1 medium head cauliflower, broken into florets
- 1 medium head broccoli, broken into florets
- 2 tablespoons vegan butter

Instructions:

1. Slice 2 of the courgettes into strips. Place on a large plate and sprinkle salt over it. Set aside for a while.
2. Slice the vegan cheese into strips of almost the same size as courgette. Set aside
3. Chop the 3rd courgette into small fine pieces.
4. Place a skillet over medium heat. Add oil. When the oil is heated, add onions and garlic and sauté until light brown. Add fine pieces of courgette and pepper and sauté until soft. Add pest. Mix well and remove from heat.

5. The courgette strips would have softened by now because of the salt.

6. Place the courgette strips on your work area. Spread the courgette filling over the strips. Place strips of vegan cheese over it. Roll it tightly and fasten with toothpicks. Place on a baking tray.

7. Sprinkle garlic over the rolls. Drizzle oil.

8. Bake in a preheated oven at 350° F for about 20- 25 minutes.

9. Meanwhile make the cauliflower and broccoli mash as follows: Steam the cauliflower and broccoli until very soft.

10. Mash the cauliflower and broccoli with a potato masher. Add vegan butter, salt and pepper and mix well.

11. Serve the rolls with mash.

Tofu with Thai Coconut Peanut Sauce

Prep: 5 min	Total: 45 min	Servings: 4-6

Ingredients:

- 8 cups mixed vegetables (keto friendly) of your choice (optional)
- ½ cup + 2 tablespoons coconut oil, divided
- 2 blocks firm tofu (around ¾ pound each)
- 6 cloves garlic, minced
- 2 shallots, finely chopped
- 2 tablespoons fresh ginger, grated
- Pepper to taste
- Salt to taste
- 4 teaspoons ground cumin
- 2/3 cup peanut butter or almond butter or cashew butter
- 2 teaspoons crushed red chili pepper
- 1 cup coconut milk
- 3 tablespoons tamari or soy sauce
- Juice of 2 limes
- 2 teaspoons vegan Thai red curry paste
- ½ cup fresh cilantro

Instructions:

1. Place the tofu over paper towels. Place a heavy bottomed skillet over it to drain excess moisture. Chop into 1-inch squares or triangles.
2. Mix together in a large dish, ½ cup oil, garlic, cumin and pepper. Add tofu slices and mix until well coated. Set aside for a while to marinate.

193

3. Place a skillet over low heat. Add oil and heat. Add shallot, ginger, crushed red chili. Cook for a few minutes until soft.
4. Add peanut butter, lime juice, coconut milk, tamari and red curry paste. Mix well and cook for 10-15 minutes. Stir a couple of times while it is cooking.
5. Add more water if you find the sauce very thick. Remove from heat and keep warm.
6. Sauté the vegetables in a pan if using with the remaining oil.
7. Place a skillet over medium heat. Add tofu mixture and cook until golden brown.
8. Place tofu with sautéed vegetables on individual serving plates. Pour sauce on top.
9. Garnish with cilantro and serve.

Vegan Cigkofte

Prep: 20 min	Total: 20 min	Servings: 4

Ingredients:

- 1 ½ cups almond flour
- 6 tablespoons ground flax
- 1 ½ cups finely ground walnuts
- 4 teaspoons paprika
- 4 teaspoons dried mint or 4 tablespoons fresh mint, finely chopped
- 4 teaspoons garlic powder or 4 cloves garlic, pressed
- 2 teaspoons dried parsley or 2 tablespoons fresh parsley, finely chopped
- ½ teaspoon pepper powder or to taste
- 1 teaspoon chili flakes
- 6 tablespoons water
- 6 tablespoons tomato puree

To serve:

- Lettuce leaves as required
- Lemon juice
- Fresh mint leaves, chopped
- Fresh parsley, chopped

Instructions:

1. Add all the ingredients into a bowl and mash using a fork until thick dough is formed. You may need to mash more until the dough is formed. It may take a while.

195

2. Take about 2 tablespoons of the dough and roll it. Place it in your fist and press lightly so that your fingers make dents in the dough. Place on a plate.
3. Repeat with the remaining dough.
4. Serve over lettuce leaves. Garnish with mint and parsley. Sprinkle lemon juice. Roll and serve.

Vegan Vegetable Moussaka

Prep: 20 min	Total: 1 hr. 20 min	Servings: 5-6

Ingredients:

For the eggplant layer:

- 4 eggplants, thinly sliced lengthwise into ¼ inch thick slices
- 4 tablespoons olive oil
- 1 tablespoon salt

For the tomato sauce:

- 5 ounces mixed nuts, finely chopped
- 2 tablespoons olive oil
- 2 tablespoons soy sauce
- 1 red bell pepper, chopped
- 1 yellow bell pepper, chopped
- 10 cloves garlic, minced

- 2 cans (14 ounces each) diced tomatoes
- ½ teaspoon ground nutmeg
- ½ teaspoon freshly ground pepper

For the almond cream:

- 1 cup almonds, soaked in water overnight, peeled
- 2 small cloves garlic
- 2 teaspoons vinegar
- ¼ teaspoons freshly ground pepper
- 1 cup water
- ¼ teaspoons salt

Instructions:

1. Sprinkle salt over the eggplant slices and place in a colander for about 30 minutes.
2. Rinse and squeeze excess moisture from the eggplants.
3. Place a parchment paper on a large baking tray. Place the eggplant slices on it in a single layer. Brush with oil.
4. Bake in a preheated oven at 390° F for about 10 minutes or until golden brown.
5. Remove from the oven and cool.
6. Meanwhile make the sauce as follows: Place a skillet over medium heat. Add all the ingredients of the sauce in it and bring to the boil.
7. Lower heat and simmer for 8-10 minutes.
8. Meanwhile make the almond cream as follows: Add all the ingredients of almond cream into a blender and blend until smooth.
9. To assemble: take a baking dish. Place alternate layers of eggplant and tomato sauce with tomato sauce as the last layer.
10. Pour almond cream on top.

11. Bake in a preheated oven at 390° F for about 25-30 minutes

Mushroom & Walnut Spicy Bolognese

Prep: 10 min	Total: 45 min	Servings: 12

Ingredients:

- 2 large onions, finely chopped
- 2 pounds mushrooms, halved, cut into fine strips
- 4 plum tomatoes, chopped
- 4 large cloves garlic, finely chopped
- 4 cans (14 ounces each) peeled, chopped tomatoes
- 2 cups walnuts, finely chopped
- 2 tablespoons tomato paste
- 4 tablespoons apple cider vinegar
- 2 tablespoons dried basil
- 2 tablespoons dried oregano
- 2 teaspoon paprika
- 2 teaspoons ground cumin
- Pepper to taste
- Salt to taste
- Red chili flakes to taste
- 4 tablespoons olive oil
- Vegan parmesan cheese to garnish

Instructions:

1. Place a saucepan over medium heat. Add oil. When the oil is heated, add onions and garlic and sauté until onions are translucent.

2. Add mushrooms and sauté for 7-8 minutes. When the moisture in the mushroom dries, add all the spices, tomato paste, vinegar, basil and oregano and mix well.
3. Add the canned and chopped tomatoes and stir.
4. Lower heat and cook for about 20 minutes. Add walnuts and cook for 5 more minutes.
5. Serve garnished with vegan Parmesan cheese.

Chapter 7: Ketogenic Vegan Dessert Recipes

Chocolate Pudding

Prep: 10 min	Total: 12 min	Servings: 6

Ingredients:

- 1 ripe avocado, peeled, pitted, chopped
- ½ cup full fat coconut milk
- ¼ cup shredded coconut
- 2 tablespoons carob powder
- 2 dried figs, chopped
- ¼ cup cocoa powder
- 2 tablespoons instant coffee
- 2 scoops plant based vanilla protein powder
- 3 tablespoons hazelnuts
- ½ teaspoon ground cinnamon
- A large pinch salt

Instructions:

1. Blend together coconut milk and avocado in a blender until smooth.
2. Add rest of the ingredients except coconut and hazelnuts. Blend until smooth.
3. Add coconut and hazelnuts and pulse for a few seconds until the hazelnut is broken into smaller pieces.
4. Transfer into serving bowls, chill and serve.

Super Easy Keto Fudge

Prep: 2 min	Total: 10 min	Servings: 4-6

Ingredients:

- 1 cup coconut butter or any other nut butter or manna
- 4 ounces sugar free chocolate or 4 ounces baker's chocolate and 30 drops stevia

Instructions:

1. Place a sheet of wax paper in a container.
2. Add chocolate and coconut butter in a pan and place the pan over low heat. Cook until well combined. Stir frequently.
3. Pour into the prepared container. Place in the refrigerator until it is set.
4. Chop into squares and serve.

Strawberry Mousse

Prep: 10 min	Total: 12 min	Servings: 12

Ingredients:

- 3 cups strawberries, sliced
- 3 cups firm tofu, drained, crumbled
- Sweetener of your choice (Swerve or stevia drops)
- A few strawberries, sliced to serve

Instructions:

1. Blend the strawberries. Add tofu and sweetener and blend until smooth.
2. Transfer into individual serving bowls and refrigerate for a few hours before serving.

Vegan Keto Sugar Cookies

Prep: 15 min	Total: 35 min	Servings: 10

Ingredients:

- 4 ounces vegan cream cheese
- 2-3 tablespoons Swerve or erythritol
- 6 tablespoons coconut flour
- ½ teaspoon almond extract
- ½ teaspoon vanilla extract

Instructions:

1. Add swerve, cream cheese, vanilla and almond extract into a bowl and beat until creamy.
2. Add coconut flour and mix to form stiff dough.
3. Place in between 2 wax papers and roll. Cut into cookies with a cookie cutter.
4. Place on a baking sheet. Bake in a preheated oven at 350° F for about 20 minutes or until the edges are golden brown in color.
5. Remove from the oven and cool completely before serving.

Vegan Ketone Gingerbread Muffin's

Prep: 20 min	Total: 40 min	Servings: 10

Ingredients:

- 2 tablespoons ground flaxseeds
- 2 tablespoons apple cider vinegar
- 4 tablespoons gingerbread spice blend
- 2 teaspoons vanilla extract
- ¾ cup almond milk or coconut milk
- 1 cup peanut butter
- 2 teaspoons baking powder
- 3-4 tablespoons swerve or to taste
- 1/8 teaspoon salt

Instructions:

1. Mix together in a bowl, flaxseeds, swerve, salt, vanilla, ginger bread spice, almond milk and set aside for 10 minutes.
2. Add peanut butter and baking powder and mix well.
3. Pour into lined muffin tins.
4. Bake in a preheated oven at 350° F for about 20 minutes or until a toothpick when inserted in the center comes out clean.
5. Cool completely before serving.

No Bake Caramel Chocolate Slice

Prep: 10 min	Total: 30 min	Servings: 4 - 6

Ingredients:

For the fudge:

- 1 cup cashew butter or any other nut butter or manna
- 4 ounces sugar free chocolate or 4 ounces baker's chocolate and 30 drops stevia
- 1 teaspoon vanilla extract
- A pinch salt
- ¾ cup almond flakes, toasted

For the chocolate layer:

- ½ cup coconut oil
- ¼ cup raw cacao powder
- 2 tablespoons swerve or maple syrup
- ¼ cup coconut milk
- 2 teaspoons vanilla extract

Instructions:

1. Place a sheet of wax paper in a container.
2. Add chocolate and coconut butter in a pan and place the pan over low heat. Cook until well combined. Stir frequently. Add vanilla and stir.

3. Pour into the prepared container. Place in the refrigerator until it is set.
4. Meanwhile, place all the ingredients except cocoa for the chocolate layer in a double boiler. When it is well blended, add cocoa powder and whisk well until smooth. Remove from heat.
5. Pour the chocolate sauce over the fudge. Spread the top with a spatula. Sprinkle the remaining almond flakes. Refrigerate for 4-5 hours before serving. Chop into squares and serve.

Mini Low Carb Peanut Butter Pumpkin Pie

Prep: 15 min	Total: 40 min	Servings: 8

Ingredients:

For the Crust:

- ½ cup coconut oil
- 2 tablespoons flaxseeds soaked in 6 tablespoons water (called flax eggs)
- ¾ cup coconut flour

For the filling:

- 2 tablespoons flaxseeds soaked in 6 tablespoons water
- ½ cup peanut butter
- ½ cup swerve or erythritol
- 1 cup pumpkin puree
- 2 teaspoons ground cinnamon

Instructions:

1. Mix together the ingredients of the crust in a bowl. Take 8 mini pie molds. Divide the mixture into the molds and press into it.
2. Mix together in a bowl all the ingredients of the filling. Divide and spread over the crust.
3. Bake in a preheated oven at 350° F for about 20 minutes.
4. Remove from the oven and cool completely before serving.

Chocolate Chia Pudding

Prep: min 10 min	Total: 45 min	Servings: 2

Ingredients:

- ½ tablespoons chia seeds
- ½ cup almond milk or soy milk, unsweetened
- ½ scoop plant based chocolate protein powder or cocoa powder
- 2 tablespoons raspberries, fresh or frozen
- ½ table spoon swerve if you are using cocoa powder

Instructions:

6. Mix together almond milk and chocolate protein powder with a whisk or fork.
7. Add chia seeds and mix well. Keep aside for 5-7 minutes. Stir again.
8. Keep aside for ½ an hour in the refrigerator.
9. Top with raspberries and serve.

Vegan Keto Protein Brownies

Prep: 15 min	Total: 40 min	Servings: 16

Ingredients:

- 3 cups warm water
- ½ cup cocoa powder, unsweetened
- 1 cup peanut butter
- ½ cup swerve or erythritol
- 4 teaspoons baking powder
- 4 scoops plant based chocolate protein powder
- ¼ cup coconut flour

Instructions:

1. Whisk together in a bowl water, swerve and peanut butter.
2. Mix together rest of the ingredients into another bowl. Add this into the peanut butter mixture and mix until well combined.
3. Pour into a greased baking dish.
4. Bake in a preheated oven at 350° F for about 20 minutes.
5. Remove from the oven and cool completely before serving.
6. Slice and serve.

Nutty Blueberry Protein Balls

Prep: 10 min	Total: 20 min	Servings: 8

Ingredients:

- 8 prunes, pitted
- 1 cup fresh strawberries, chopped
- 1 cup macadamia nuts, unsalted, roasted
- 2 cups walnuts or almonds
- 1 cup shredded coconut, unsweetened
- 4 tablespoons coconut oil, melted

Instructions:

1. Place the prunes in the food processor bowl and pulse until smooth.
2. Add walnuts or almonds and macadamia nuts. Pulse until the nuts are finely chopped.
3. With the food processor running, slowly pour melted coconut oil. Let the food processor run until the mixture is well combined.
4. Transfer the mixture into a bowl. Add strawberries and mix well to form dough. Shape the dough into small balls.
5. Place the shredded coconut on a plate. Roll the balls in the shredded coconut and place on another plate.
6. Refrigerate the balls until ready to serve. Keep the unused ones refrigerated in an airtight container. It can last for 4-5 days when refrigerated.

Chocolate Peanut Butter Low Carb Vegan Ice Cream

Prep: 15 min	Total: 17 min + freezing time	Servings: 8 -12

Ingredients:

- 4 large Hass avocadoes, peeled, pitted, chopped
- ½ cup peanut butter
- ½ cup cacao powder, unsweetened
- 20 drops stevia drops or to taste

Instructions:

1. Add all the ingredients into a blender and blend until smooth. Pour into a freezer safe container and freeze for 4-5 hours or until set.
2. Scoop and serve.

Fresh Strawberry Lime Popsicles

Prep: 10 min	Total: 12 min + freezing time	Servings: 5 - 6

Ingredients:

- 20 medium to large strawberries
- Zest of 2 limes
- ¼ cup water

Instructions:

1. Add all the ingredients into a blender and blend until smooth.
2. Pour into Popsicle moulds and freeze.
3. Remove from mould and serve.

Conclusion

I thank you once again for choosing this book and hope you had a good time reading it. The main aim of this book was to teach you the basics of the ketogenic diet and give you simple recipes.

All the recipes are tried and tested and sure to leave you smacking your lips. However, do not limit yourself to just these and come up with some of your own.

You can freely mix up the menu and switch between the lunch and dinner recipes. You can also switch up the ingredients and come up with interesting dishes.

Remember that the ketogenic is not a fad diet and will require you to turn it into a lifestyle choice. Once you get started with it, you will have to make the effort to stick with it for life.

I hope you have the chance to avail all the benefits provided by the diet!

Good luck!